Professional Communication
in Audiology

Professional Communication in Audiology

Virginia Ramachandran, AuD, PhD
Brad A. Stach, PhD

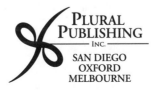

PLURAL
PUBLISHING
INC.

SAN DIEGO
OXFORD
MELBOURNE

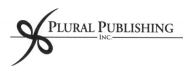

5521 Ruffin Road
San Diego, CA 92123

e-mail: info@pluralpublishing.com
Web site: http://www.pluralpublishing.com

FSC
www.fsc.org
MIX
Paper from
responsible sources
FSC® C011935

Typeset in 11/13 Garamond by Flanagan's Publishing Services, Inc.
Printed in the United States of America by McNaughton & Gunn

Library of Congress Cataloging-in-Publication Data

Ramachandran, Virginia, author.
  Professional communication in audiology / Virginia Ramachandran, Brad A.
Stach.
      pages ; cm
  Includes bibliographical references and index.
  ISBN-13: 978-1-59756-365-9 (alk. paper)
  ISBN-10: 1-59756-365-X (alk. paper)
  I. Stach, Brad A., author. II. Title.
  [DNLM: 1. Audiology. 2. Communication. 3. Professional-Patient Relations.
WV 270]
  RF290
  617.80023—dc23
                                                    2013006757

Contents

Introduction

The ability to communicate with patients, families, and other professionals is a critical component of clinical practice. No matter how capable clinicians might be at performing diagnostic testing, interpreting results, and formulating appropriate interventions, any failure to communicate results and recommendations effectively reduces the optimum value of the services provided.

Effective communication must be achieved throughout the assessment process to obtain and convey necessary information. For example, without appropriate instruction, patients may not understand the purpose of tests or how to correctly participate in them. Effective communication must also occur to formulate treatment and management options. If patients and families do not understand test results and the impact of hearing loss on communication, they may not understand the disorder or need for intervention.

The communicative competence necessary for successful clinical practice extends to both verbal and written abilities. Clinicians simply must be able to talk and write effectively.

This book provides communication strategies specific to the context of clinical evaluation and treatment in audiology. It is not intended as an exhaustive summary of the underlying basic skills of verbal and written communication. Such issues are effectively dealt with in other texts. Rather than focusing on the basics of how to communicate, this text focuses on audiologic communication—what to communicate and how.

Everybody thinks they are right about their views on communicating with patients and other healthcare providers. We (the authors) are no different. This text contains a summary of our perspectives on communicating with patients and providers. Where evidence is available to base these opinions, it is provided. Unfortunately, in the clinical world, there is not always a solid evidence base upon which to draw. In those cases, we humbly rely on our clinical experience, which is necessarily colored by our practice setting—a large hospital system with a heavy emphasis on diagnostics, where we communicate with a myriad of physicians and other providers via a relatively sophisticated electronic health record system.

Your practice situation may differ. Although it is not our intent to ignore other types of practice settings, we base our thoughts and perspectives on the health care arena and, where we can, try to generalize them to the larger context.

Professional Communication in Audiology is designed to provide beginning clinicians and students with perspective and instruction in the art and science of verbal and written communication in the clinical setting. Chapter 1 provides an overview of the factors and influences that guide the practice of clinical communication. Part I covers the clinical application of verbal communication with patients and families. Part II addresses documentation and written communication for other providers.

A number of individuals have assisted in the process of creating this book. We are particularly appreciative of the efforts of all of those at Plural Publishing who have guided us through the publishing process. It is our sincere hope that instructors and students will find the material in this book helpful in their quest for translating theoretical material into clinical skills.

We dedicate this book in loving memory of Dr. Sadanand Singh.

"How lucky I am to have something that
makes saying goodbye so hard."

—A.A. Milne

CHAPTER 1

What Guides Professional Communication?

When considering how to communicate in clinical situations, it is reasonable to wonder "Who decides how I should communicate as a professional?" There are numerous factors and influences that guide the practice of clinical report writing and communication with patients, and no one source provides definitive answers on how to communicate in the clinical world. Considerations regarding research evidence for best practice, reimbursement, professional standards, and the administrative milieu in which one practices all contribute to the manner in which professional communication is implemented. Ultimately, the professional must weigh the various factors to determine how to best serve the needs of the patient and providers. Table 1–1 summarizes factors that may impact communication decisions.

Research Evidence

Where evidence exists to guide practice, it should be used to make appropriate choices for communication. For example, review of research in communication in medical care demonstrates that the use of professional interpreters for patients with limited English proficiency improves outcomes for comprehension, utilization of health care services, patient outcomes, and patient satisfaction,

1

Table 1–1. Factors That Impact Communication Decisions

1. Research evidence
2. Employer guidelines
3. Third-party provider expectations
4. Accrediting bodies
5. Laws and regulations
6. The professional

compared to the use of ad hoc interpreters (Karliner, 2007). Evidence such as this should be used to guide decisions regarding clinical communication strategies.

Employer Guidelines

In some cases, institutions or settings in which an audiologist practices provide guidelines for communication within the setting. Settings most likely to have guidelines for documentation and reporting include school systems, government agencies, and major medical systems. In cases where there are numerous providers and a large patient caseload, uniformity of reporting assists in the effectiveness of the communication process. Institutional guidelines may also reflect philosophies for best practice established by the facility. In cases where such guidelines exist, it is important to be aware of and to follow guidelines for optimal patient care.

Third-Party Providers

Another important consideration in documentation and reporting is the third-party payer for medical services. In cases where patients have health care insurance, documentation and reporting are typically designed to accommodate the demands of third-party payers. These document demands pertain to what was done for a patient and why. Accommodating third-party payer stipulations for documentation is likely to maximize the potential for appropriate reimbursement of services. As an example, Blue Cross–Blue Shield of

Michigan (BCBSM) has a provider manual for documentation guidelines. The stated purpose of the guidelines is to "determine that the services, procedures and devices billed . . . were provided in accordance with the provisions of your participation agreement," and to ensure that the procedures were "medically necessary, ordered by the physician, provided to the patient, and documented in the medical record" (BCBSM, 2005). Medical records may be audited by insurance providers to determine whether services that were billed meet these criteria. If they do not, the insurer may seek to recover payment from providers whose documentation does not meet the guidelines. A list of the guidelines for information to be included by providers for this particular insurer is shown is Table 1–2.

Table 1–2. General Guidelines for Medical Record Documentation — BCBSM

Identifying Information

- Patient's name and address
- Patient's contract and group numbers
- Patient's date of birth
- Patient's gender
- Physician's name and address
- Facility's name and address
- Location where services are provided

Patient Encounter

- Chief complaint and relevant history, including all pertinent health risks
- Pertinent physical examination findings and prior diagnostic test results
- Patient's progress, response to and changes in treatment, and revision of diagnosis
- Assessment, clinical impression, or diagnosis
- Plan for care

Medical Record Entry

- Date and time and information are documented
- Signature or initials of individual documenting
- Credentials of providers (e.g., AuD)

Accrediting Bodies

In the field of audiology and in health care generally, there are various accrediting bodies helping to standardize care and set expectations for health care service. Such accrediting bodies typically issue guidelines to help the professional communicate effectively.

The Joint Commission on Accreditation of Healthcare Organizations (JCAHO or Joint Commission) is a private, nonprofit organization that provides accreditation to health care organizations and hospitals in an effort to ensure certain requirements for patient safety and quality of care are met. Hospitals receiving payment from the U.S. federal health care programs, Center for Medicare and Medicaid Services (CMS), must be accredited by the Joint Commission. As part of its mission to improve safety and the quality of health care to the public, the Joint Commission has standards for communication in health care settings between the provider and patient and among providers. The guiding principle of the Joint Commission's communication guidelines is based on the idea that "effective communication is a cornerstone of patient safety" (The Joint Commission, 2007).

The Joint Commission has developed a communication guide for increasing effectiveness of provider communication with patients. Among a host of methods for optimizing communication, The Joint Commission advises that:

❖ "teach-back" and "show-back" techniques, wherein the patient demonstrates to the provider that information conveyed has been understood, be used to ensure patient comprehension of information;

❖ providers speak slowly and in plain language to patients;

❖ information provided to patients be limited to two or three main points;

❖ at least two identifiers be used to verify the identity of a patient to prevent mistakes (The Joint Commission, 2007);

❖ providers adhere to an official "Do Not Use" list of abbreviations (The Joint Commission, 2009) to minimize errors in interpreting written communications (examples of abbreviations that are discouraged from being used by providers are shown in Table 1–3);

Table 1–3. Joint Commission "Do Not Use" List

Do Not Use	Use Instead
U (unit)	Write "unit"
IU (international unit)	Write "international unit"
Q.D., QD, q.d., qd (daily)	Write "daily"
Q.O.D., QOD, q.o.d., qod (every other day)	Write "every other day"
Trailing zero (X.0 mg)	Write X mg
Lack of leading zero (.X mg)	Write 0.X mg
MS, MSO_4, and $MgSO_4$	Write "morphine sulfate" or "magnesium sulfate"

Additional Abbreviations, Acronyms, and Symbols

Do Not Use	Use Instead
> (greater than)	Write "greater than"
< (less than)	Write "less than"
Abbreviations for drug names	Write drug names in full
Apothecary units	Use metric units
@	Write "at"
cc	Write "mL" or "ml" or "milliliters"
µg	Write "mcg" or "micrograms"

❖ providers adopt a universal "time out" protocol to verify accuracy of information with all involved providers prior to initiating a procedure, in an effort to minimize the potential for procedures on patients to be performed at the wrong site, on the incorrect patient, or using an incorrect procedure; and

❖ providers participate in research initiatives examining methods to improve patient care and safety for culturally and linguistically diverse patient populations (The Joint Commission, 2010; Wilson-Stronks & Galvez, 2007; Wilson-Stronks, Lee, Cordero, Kopp, & Galvez, 2008).

Note that the terms in the Joint Commission "do not use" list generally apply to providers other than audiologists. Audiologists often use profession-specific jargon and abbreviations. Most patients and providers are unfamiliar with these abbreviations, and use of them will likely result in confusion. Of interest to audiologists, Canada's Institute for Safe Mediation Practices includes prohibitions against the use of "AD" for "right ear," "AS" for "left ear," and "AU" for "each ear or both ears." Audiologists should use full terms when writing, rather than abbreviations. Examples of such terms are included in Table 1–4.

Laws and Regulations

There are numerous federal laws that address communication issues as they relate to the civil rights of individuals and equal access to services. Generally, these laws apply to organizations that receive federal funding. Hospitals and other health care providers

Table 1–4. Audiology "Do Not Use" List

Do Not Use	Use Instead
AU	Both, bilaterally
AS	Left
AD	Right
SNHL	Sensorineural hearing loss
CHL	Conductive hearing loss
HL	Hearing loss
WRS	Word recognition score
SRT	Speech recognition threshold
Tymp	Tympanogram
HA	Hearing aid
ABR	Auditory brainstem response
VNG	Videonystagmography

typically receive federal funding via the CMS programs (Medicare and Medicaid) and federal research grants, making them subject to these laws. These laws may affect aspects of how audiologists communicate with patients.

Title VI of the Civil Rights Act of 1964 prohibits discrimination of individuals on the basis of race, color, or national origin by any program receiving federal assistance. This act has been interpreted to mean that individuals with limited English proficiency may be considered to be discriminated against on the basis of national origin if efforts are not made to provide equitable access to services. Typically, access to services is accomplished through the use of professional interpreters and translation of written documents into languages often encountered in the community of the health care institution. To comply with this law, audiologists should utilize professional interpreters when communicating with patients whose preferred language for medical communication is not English. Professionally translated documents should also be utilized to communicate written information.

There are at least two laws applicable to communication with individuals who are deaf or hard of hearing. Section 504 of the Rehabilitation Act of 1973 is enforced by the Health and Human Services Office for Civil Rights. This law prohibits discrimination against individuals with disabilities, including hearing loss, by any program receiving federal assistance. The Americans with Disabilities Act is enforced by the Department of Justice. This law requires that institutions receiving federal assistance provide public accommodations to individuals with disabilities to ensure access to participation. Both laws require that hospitals provide auxiliary aids to individuals with disabilities when necessary to ensure effective communication. Such services may include the use of qualified interpreters and hearing-assistive technology.

Other federal, state, and local laws may also address issues of communication in the medical setting, and it is important to be aware of how such laws may impact the audiologist's decisions regarding communication with patients.

The Professional

Last and most important, professionals are personally responsible for developing appropriate and useful methods for both verbal and written communication. It is their responsibility to formulate intelligent and thoughtful strategies for communication. The ultimate goals for patient encounters and interactions with other providers must guide the strategies used for maximally effective communication.

❖ The Importance of Privacy ❖

Trust is one of the most important qualities of the relationship between a patient and health care provider. One aspect of this relationship is the unmitigated expectation that providers will not divulge patients' personal information. Breaches of this trust are one of the most serious errors a professional can make. Violations of laws designed to protect health care information can result in substantial fines and even imprisonment. Without confidence in the ability to trust health care providers with information, patients may be reluctant or unwilling to disclose information or to seek health care, even when absolutely necessary. This may pose significant and serious risk to themselves and others. A patient has every right to expect that health care providers will not share private information. Audiologists have the responsibility to guard and protect the personal and confidential information of their patients.

Professional Ethics and Privacy

Health care professionals often belong to organizations representing their profession. Most professional associations have a code of ethics. The code of ethics serves to guide professional behavior and decision making, protect the rights of consumers, and instill a sense of trust in the public whom the professionals serve. Professional organizations often have methods for censure of members who violate codes of ethical conduct, including sanctions up to the revocation of membership as the maximum punishment.

In the profession of audiology, there are several large national organizations that have traditionally acted as representatives of the audiology profession. Among them are the American Academy of Audiology (AAA), the American Speech-Language-Hearing Association (ASHA), and the Academy of Doctors of Audiology (ADA). All of these organizations have a Code of Ethics that contains statements regarding or relating to protection of personal information.

The Code of Ethics of the American Academy of Audiology has as its first principle, "Members shall provide professional services and conduct research with honesty and compassion, and shall respect the dignity, worth, and rights of those served." Privacy and protection of personal information are included in the concept of respect for the patient. Principle 3 of the Code states that, "Members shall maintain the confidentiality of the information and records of those receiving services or involved in research." The associated Rule 3a directs that "Individuals shall not reveal to unauthorized persons any professional or personal information obtained from the person served professionally, unless required by law."

The American Speech-Language-Hearing Association Code of Ethics states as its first principle of ethics that "Individuals shall honor their responsibility to hold paramount the welfare of persons they serve professionally or participants in research and scholarly activities . . . ." An associated ethical rule instructs that "Individuals shall not reveal, without authorization, any professional or personal information about identified persons, served professionals, or identified participants involved in research and scholarly activities unless required by law to do so, or unless doing so is necessary to protect the welfare of the person or of the community or otherwise required by law."

The Academy of Doctors of Audiology has as its No. 1 principle of ethics "to protect the welfare of persons served professionally." Rule 5 of this principle states that "Members shall not release professional and personal information obtained from the patient without the written permission of the patient in accordance with applicable state and federal law."

All of these codes of ethics clearly spell out the ethical obligation of audiologists to maintain patient confidentiality in order to protect patients.

HIPAA

Another important consideration of privacy in health care is the Health Insurance Portability and Accountability Act (HIPAA). HIPAA is federal legislation that was enacted in 1996. This legislation was enacted for two major purposes. The first purpose, covered by Title I of HIPAA, is to protect health insurance coverage for individuals and their families who change or lose employment. The second purpose, covered by Title II of HIPAA, is to establish national standards for transactions involving electronic health care records and to establish a system of national identifiers for health care providers. It is this second portion of HIPAA, also known as the Administration Simplification provisions, that is particularly relevant to audiologic practice.

The HIPAA rules define those health care providers known as "covered entities" who are held to the standards set forth by the legislation. Audiologists, as health care providers, are accountable to the guidelines set forth in the legislation.

Title II of HIPAA charges the Department of Health and Human Services (HHS) with development of rules to realize the goal of increasing efficiency in health care through the use of standardized practices for use and dissemination of health care information. Five rules have been created by HHS to fulfill this mission. These rules are: the Transactions and Code Sets Rule, the Unique Identifiers Rule, the Privacy Rule, the Security Rule, and the Enforcement Rule. These components are outlined in Table 1–5.

The Transactions and Code Sets Rule refers to the need for providers who electronically file claims with the CMS to file claims using HIPAA standards for electronic information. This rule impacts audiologists to the extent that they utilize electronic means for transmitting patient health care data such as billing of services to CMS.

The National Provider Identifier Rule mandates that health care providers using electronic transfer of medical information have a National Provider Identifier (NPI) number. Audiologists working in facilities with electronic transfer of information, such as for billing purposes, must have an NPI.

The Privacy Rule regulates the use and disclosure of what is known as Protected Health Information (PHI). Protected health information consists broadly of information that can be linked to a particular individual and includes health status, provision of health care, and payment for health care. The information typically covered includes any part of an individual's medical record or payment history and can exist in any format, including on paper, electroni-

Table 1–5. HIPAA Components

Title I: Health care access, portability, and renewability

Title II: Preventing health care fraud and abuse; administrative simplification; medical liability reform

- Privacy rule
- Transactions and code sets rule
- Security rule
- Unique identifiers rule (National Provider Identifier)
- Enforcement rule

cally, or orally. HIPAA narrowly defines patient identifiers as a list of 18 different pieces of information that can be used to link the identity of individuals with their health care information (Centers for Disease Control and Prevention, 2003). These identifiers are listed in Table 1–6.

The Privacy Rule generally prevents providers from disclosing protected health information, except in particular circumstances. It also mandates that when information is disclosed, only the minimum necessary information is provided. Circumstances under which information may be disclosed include the need to facilitate treatment, payment, or health care operations, or when authorization is obtained from the individual. There are provisions for providing nonauthorized PHI in specific situations for mandated reporting, such as suspected child abuse, neglect, and other circumstances. The Privacy Rule mandates that health care providers inform patients of documented privacy policies and procedures. Providers must also maintain records of disclosure of health care information. Covered entities must appoint a Privacy Official, who is responsible for administration of the rules, and a contact person, who manages complaints and training of all members of the staff regarding privacy rules (Centers for Disease Control and Prevention, 2003).

Table 1–6. Personal Health Information Identifiers

1. Names.

2. All geographic subdivisions smaller than a state, including street address, city, county, precinct, ZIP code, and their equivalent geocodes, except for the initial three digits of a ZIP code if, according to the current publicly available data from the Bureau of Census, (1) the geographic units formed by combining all ZIP codes with the same three initial digits contain more than 20,000 people, and (2) the initial three digits of a ZIP code for all such geographic units containing 20,000 or fewer people are changed to 000.

3. All elements of dates (except year) for dates directly related to the individual, including birth date, admission date, discharge date, date of death, and all ages over 89 and all elements of dates (including year) indicative of such age, except that such ages and elements may be aggregated into a single category of age 90 or older.

4. Telephone numbers.

5. Fax numbers.

6. Electronic mail addresses.

7. Social Security numbers.

8. Medical record numbers.

9. Health plan beneficiary numbers.

10. Account numbers.

11. Certificate/license numbers.

12. Vehicle identifiers and serial numbers, including license plate numbers.

13. Device identifiers and serial numbers.

14. Web Universal Resource Locators (URLs).

15. Internet Protocol (IP) address numbers.

16. Biometric identifiers, including finger and voice prints.

17. Full-face photographic images and any comparable images.

18. Any other unique identifying number, characteristic, or code, except as permitted for reidentification purposes provided certain conditions are met. In addition to the removal of the above-stated identifiers, the covered entity may not have actual knowledge that the remaining information could be used alone or in combination with any other information to identify an individual who is the subject of the information.

The Privacy Rule has numerous implications for audiologic practice and research. Clinicians must limit disclosure of information. When it is necessary to disclose information, only the minimal amount of information needed for provision of care should be provided. For example, if a patient is to be contacted and told that a hearing aid is back from repair, and a message is left on voice-mail, only the information necessary for the patient to return the phone call should be shared. Additional information regarding the purpose of the contact should remain private.

When information needs to be shared, authorization should be obtained from the patient. A "Release of Information" form can be used to document the patient's authorization of disclosure of health information. For example, a clinician may wish to communicate with a child's teacher about strategies for successful listening in the classroom. The audiologist must first obtain authorization from the patient's legal guardian to discuss the child's hearing health care information with the teacher.

Overall, reasonable efforts should be made in all patient encounters and with patient records to maintain the confidentiality and privacy of health information. In many cases, patients are accompanied by other family members or friends. It is appropriate to communicate with others when authorized by the patient to do so. Information that is shared with others should be limited to that which is necessary to assist the patient in provision of health care. For example, an adult child of a patient seen for an audiologic evaluation may be provided with information regarding the results of the test and may be involved in treatment planning, so long as the family member is involved in the care of the patient and the patient assents.

The Security Rule has similar goals to the Privacy Rule for protection of patient information, but it deals specifically with protection of electronic health information. The Security Rule mandates administrative, physical, and technical safeguards for protecting electronic PHI. These safeguards include having plans for the protection of information: restricting physical access to equipment where electronic medical information is stored, using technological means to restrict access to electronic medical information to those who should not access it, and ensuring that information transmitted is done so in a manner that keeps it secure and protected.

One example of a technical safeguard is the use of passwords for accessing electronic medical information. Electronic equipment used by audiologists that includes storage of patient data should comply with HIPAA standards for protecting patient information.

The Enforcement Rule is meant to provide a means for enforcement of HIPAA rules by creating penalties for rules violations.

Concern for Privacy as a Guide to Clinical Behavior

What confidentiality standards mean for the clinical world is that information that does not have an absolute need to be shared should not be discussed, even with other professionals. When such information does need to be shared, it should be done so in a manner that is least likely to allow patient information to be accidentally exposed to other individuals. For example, when talking about a particular case with a colleague, the discussion must be done in a professional manner. The audiologist should address the patient's information with other professionals in the same manner that would occur if the patient were present and listening to the conversation. Such consultations and discussions should occur in discreet locations, where individuals not involved in the case are unable to overhear personal information.

When information must be transferred outside of the audiologist's office, or otherwise shared with other professionals, it is necessary for the patient to provide permission for the transfer of information. The most common method of providing permission is through the use of a "Release of Information" document wherein terms are explicitly stated for who may disclose information, what type of information may be disclosed, and to whom disclosure may be made.

Without such permission, the audiologist has a responsibility to maintain as private any information about the patient. Frequently in our profession, there are other family members involved in patient care, such as children or spouses, who request information regarding evaluation outcomes and audiologic intervention recommendations. This information should be shared with others, including family members, only when the patient has provided permission to do so.

PART I

Verbal Communication with Patients

CHAPTER 2

Audiologist as a Communicator: Knowing Your Communication Partner

Audiology is a care-based profession, meaning, of course, that it is focused on people. Our patients are the reason we do what we do. In order to communicate with our patients and to be of help to them, we first have to understand them and their unique experience. Lao Tzu, the ancient Chinese philosopher, said, "Knowing others is intelligence; knowing yourself is true wisdom." This chapter will focus on the truth of the first part of this statement (leaving the latter for your own personal existential journey). In this chapter we will discuss building rapport, culture competence, and overcoming barriers to communication.

❖ Ensuring the Correct Patient ❖

It may seem obvious that it is important to ensure that the patient with whom you are talking is, in fact, the patient to whom you are intending to talk. Remarkably, it is not an uncommon occurrence in medical settings for the identity of patients to be confused. Patients may mistakenly believe that they have been called from the waiting area, and this is probably more likely to occur in a population of individuals who do not hear well, such as those seen by audiologists. It is recommended that at least two personal identifiers be used to verify that the patient being seen is the correct one. It is not uncommon to ask the patient's name and date of birth to confirm the correct identity of the patient.

❖ Building Rapport ❖

When first meeting a patient and family, regardless of the type of audiologic encounter, the first goal is to establish a positive working relationship. The first moments of meeting the patient can set the tone for the remainder of the encounter and can easily facilitate or interfere with communication with the patient or family.

The establishment of rapport with a patient and family members begins with greetings and introductions. Most patients appreciate being addressed by a formal title, such as Mr. or Ms. If the patient is accompanied by others, it is important and proper to determine the relationship of the others to the patient. Audiologists should introduce themselves using their name and appropriate title, as well as those of any students or observers. They should inform the patient of what will take place during the encounter and how long the evaluation or appointment will take. Table 2–1 provides a simple framework for recalling the various steps in establishing a positive relationship with the patient, using the convenient acronym AIDET.

In addition to choosing a language level that is appropriate to the patient, the manner in which those words are spoken conveys a message to the patient of the clinician's attitudes and state

Table 2–1. The AIDET Strategy for Patient Encounters

Acknowledge the patient via greeting, eye contact, shaking hands, and so forth

Introduce yourself to the patient and identify your role

Duration—provide the patient with an estimate of the amount of time the encounter will take

Expectation—inform the patient of what to expect during the encounter

Thank the patient

---

of mind. A warm smile and a handshake upon meeting go a long way toward creating a comfortable and welcoming environment to the patient. It is important that the tone conveyed to the patient be one of empathy and open-mindedness. Patients will present from a variety of backgrounds and cultural milieus, as well as with various temporary or chronic conditions that can impact state of mind and mood. Some patients will arrive on time with smiles on their faces, and others will not. Nevertheless, it is important for patients to have the opportunity to gain trust as the health care provider seeks to understand the patient's condition. In doing so, it is often necessary to seek information about a variety of personal issues the patient may not be immediately prepared to share. Verbal and nonverbal behaviors of the provider will help shape rapport with the patient and will impact the patient's response to these helping efforts. Even if a patient presents with an unpleasant attitude or displays hostile emotions, the audiologist must remain neutral and professional in interactions to diffuse negative attitudes to the extent possible and to provide an avenue for the patient to share necessary information.

When evaluating children, the audiologist is more likely to obtain important and necessary information if rapport is established prior to testing. One way to make children feel included in the session and to initially build rapport with the child is to bend down or kneel to greet them at eye level. When testing older children it is often helpful to address the child directly when asking case history questions and filling in missing information from the caregiver as needed. When counseling regarding test results, it is important to engage the child, as appropriate, to explain results. It is also helpful to directly address older children when providing information about the hearing test outcomes and to emphasize approval of their performance during behavioral testing.

❖ Understanding the Communicative Partner ❖

Understanding the communicative partner as an individual is a necessary step in communicating with the patient and in gaining the knowledge necessary to provide effective assessment and recommendations to the patient for his or her particular hearing and balance problems. The audiologist brings knowledge of hearing and balance to the process, but this knowledge must be utilized in the context of the patient's unique personal experience. Factors such as language and culture impact the communication process. In addition, other factors such as previous experience with audiologists, hearing loss that impacts ability to communicate effectively with the provider, maladaptive communication strategies, and cognitive challenges will impact the communication process as well. It is necessary for the audiologist to understand and appreciate these factors in order to facilitate effective communication with the patient.

Cultural competence refers to the ability to effectively address the needs of individuals of diverse cultures (The Joint Commission, 2010). This includes: (a) valuing diversity, (b) self-assessment as it relates to cultural competence, (c) managing differences, (d) acquiring knowledge of other cultures, and (e) adapting to the cultures of the communities served by the health care provider.

For example, the authors' home area (Detroit, Michigan) has one of the largest Arab populations outside of the Middle East. Providers who practice in this area must be cognizant of the influences that this culture may bring to the health care setting. In addition to language differences, there are socioeconomic factors, familial and gender relationships, and religious traditions, including dietary restrictions, which may be important in the health care setting. The cultural context may also influence how patients respond to diagnosis and treatment suggestions. In cultural traditions where the extended family is of utmost importance, such as in the Arab culture, diagnosis of hearing loss in an infant can bring the additional burden of reflecting poorly on the family in the community, as this may be perceived as a genetic weakness inherent in the family (Hammad, Kysia, Rahab, Hassoun, & Connelly, 1999). Awareness of this type of response is obviously important in helping to counsel the family about hearing loss.

❖ Uniqueness of Patients ❖

Communication is not a one-size-fits-all activity. When it comes to diagnostic evaluation, patients generally want the same information: presence and nature of the disorder, recommendations, and prognosis for audiologic intervention. Insofar as patients are in search of the same general information, communication goals are similar. However, differences between and within these groups will determine more specific information being sought and the level of understanding that can be assumed when communicating.

The example described in the previous section also demonstrates the diversity inherent in different cultural communities. The "Arab-American" community of the Detroit area includes people from a wide range of countries of origin, religions, socioeconomic status, and political experiences. Whereas it may be necessary to understand the common experiences and expectations of the cultural community that you serve, it is equally important to understand that each patient and family is unique, and it is important to avoid stereotyping patients. Each patient and family should be regarded as individuals, and an open mind should be assumed regarding appropriate patient care. The balance of these two issues can be summed up as follows: Each new patient encounter should be approached by the provider as an opportunity to learn about a patient's particular cultural needs, but each provider should be prepared with a basis of knowledge for what those needs might be to facilitate appropriate patient care.

Most patients have scant knowledge of the structure or function of the ear. They have little to no idea what to expect in terms of testing or what to expect in terms of outcomes and recommendations. It is necessary in such cases to inform the patient of what to expect during the evaluation. These patients will also benefit most from the use of easily understood language and concepts to describe outcomes and how they characterize structure or function of the auditory system. The description of the degree of hearing loss will be most readily understood when described in terms of communication function. The patient will also benefit from accurate and consistent terminology to describe the nature of the hearing loss.

Some patients, however, have a deeper understanding of the concepts being measured during the evaluation. Often musicians, engineers, physicians who are patients, patients with long-standing hearing loss, and others may have sufficient experience or knowledge to express more interest in the details of the testing and the specific acoustic consequences of their hearing loss. These patients typically require more extensive and in-depth counseling. It is important to approach each patient individually and to assess the extent and manner in which information should be presented.

❖ Barriers to Communication ❖

Audiologists may occasionally discover substantial barriers to effective communication with patients and families. Examples of such barriers may include the effect of the hearing loss, patients and families who speak a different language, people who have other communication difficulties, and extremely talkative patients.

Hearing Loss

In communicating with individuals with potential hearing loss it is important to use communication strategies that help facilitate understanding of speech. It is typically necessary to modify speaking style to speak clearer and slower than usual. It is also helpful for most patients to be able to see the provider's face while listening so that they can utilize visual cues to better understand. For some patients, these measures are insufficient, and some sort of amplification device or talking via headphones is useful for facilitating communication. Writing is an option when these methods are insufficient.

Communicating in the Patient's Language

In the health care setting, communication is a vital aspect of diagnosis and treatment. Differences in language use between provider and patient may result in impoverished care. Research has demonstrated evidence of health care disparities for individuals from minority cultures, particularly language-minority cultures (Wilson-Stronks et al., 2008). The ability to communicate with patients in their language is not only a patient right, it is necessary for quality care.

In addition to improving quality of care, making language interpretation services available is necessary to satisfy legal and regulatory requirements. As discussed in Chapter 1, laws such as Title VI of the Civil Rights Act of 1964 mandate that language services must be provided to patients who have limited English proficiency.

Numerous resources have been developed to understand and respond to the language needs of patients in health care settings.

The Office of Minority Health of the U.S. Department of Health and Human Services (2001) has published standards for culturally and linguistically appropriate services in health care. Based on these recommendations, The Joint Commission (Wilson-Stronks & Galvez, 2007) collected data on how health systems in the United States were, in fact, meeting the needs of patients with additional language and cultural needs. This was followed by a framework for establishing practices to meet the needs of diverse populations and a self-assessment tool for health systems to use when determining their own ability to meet patient needs (Wilson-Stronks et al., 2008). In 2010, The Joint Commission published a "roadmap" for health systems to plan for meeting patient needs, including suggestions for how to meet current and proposed Joint Commission standards relating to the communication and cultural needs of patients.

One of the most commonly used methods for communicating with patients who have limited English proficiency is the use of professional interpreters. Professional interpreters are distinguished from ad hoc interpreters such as family members, friends, and others. Professional interpreters are different from these other groups in that they are trained in the performance of interpretation. In particular, professional medical interpreters are trained to understand often complex medical terminology and how to communicate effectively with patients in the medical setting. The use of ad hoc interpreters should be avoided. Individuals who are not trained to provide interpretation services may do an inadequate job interpreting medical information. Family members and friends may not always relay correct information to the patient for various reasons. In particular, the use of children as interpreters should be avoided, as they are less likely to possess the emotional or cognitive maturity necessary to interpret medical issues. Research literature in this area demonstrates that the use of professional interpreters is associated with improved clinical care for patients with limited English proficiency when compared to the use of ad hoc interpreters (Karliner et al., 2007).

Interpreters may be available in person or by other means, such as video conferencing, or more typically, by telephone. When possible, arranging for such services prior to the appointment can save a great deal of time.

The Association of American Medical Colleges offers guidelines for the use of medical interpreter services. Following assessment of the need for an interpreter and the procurement of services, the medical interpreter should be briefed about the goals of the patient contact. The interpreter should be asked to interpret in a conduit fashion, meaning that there is literal interpretation in the first person, with no omissions, editing, polishing, or outside conversation. When using an interpreter, face and speak directly to the patient, making eye contact and speaking in the first person. The use of an interpreter during the patient encounter should also be documented in the patient's medical record. A list of tips on speaking to patients via language interpreters can be found in Table 2–2.

The process of interpretation, which is the conversion of spoken language from one language to another, is different than translation, the conversion of written language from one language to another. The skill sets necessary for interpretation and translation are different, and interpreters should not be asked to translate written documents on sight.

Other Concerns
(Cognitive, Speech/Language Deficits, etc.)

Some patients may have difficulty providing or receiving information. Examples include very young patients, patients who have difficulty with speech production, and patients who have cogni-

Table 2–2. Tips for Speaking to Patients via Language Interpreters

---

- Keep sentences short

- Use simple language

- Avoid asking more than one question at a time

- Avoid slang or technical terms

- Pause often to allow the interpreter to speak

- Speak directly to the patient

- Document the use of interpreter services in the medical record

---

tive issues that impact communication. It is important that case history and recommendations be tailored accordingly. In terms of language, modifications to typical words chosen may be needed. Most patients will not have previous knowledge of the auditory system or hearing and will need explanations to be presented as clearly and simply as possible to promote greatest understanding. Patients who are elderly or sick may tire easily, and brevity in such situations will be an important ally.

Time Constraints

In some cases, the audiologist may encounter patients who talk excessively. In many cases, such patients may simply have a great deal of information to convey, and allowing the patient to talk about concerns in an open-ended fashion may accomplish the same outcomes as asking questions of the patient. However, in some cases, overly talkative patients may be exhibiting maladaptive communication strategies. Some patients may find that by dominating a communication interaction, they are better able to control the conversation to more effectively hear and understand what is being said with their hearing loss. Such communication strategies often cause a barrier to communication, as the clinician may be unable to elicit or provide necessary information. In this case, the most successful strategy will be to provide the patient with structure regarding the type of information that needs to be elicited or provided. This way the patient is prepared to hear certain information and may become more relaxed about communicating because the subject of the interaction is known. It is also appropriate to mention to the patient when necessary that there is a lot of information that must be covered during the appointment. The goals for the appointment should be emphasized so that the patient is aware of what to expect and attends to the subject of conversation. The patient can also be rescheduled for an additional appointment in the future if it is necessary to do so.

CHAPTER 3

Audiologist as Detective: Gathering Evidence

Prior to initiating contact with a patient, the audiologist should have a goal for the encounter and a plan for how to reach that goal. For diagnostic testing, the goals should include: (a) obtaining information relevant to the presenting concern, (b) obtaining information about the patient's symptoms and audiologic history, (c) communicating instructions about evaluation to obtain appropriate results, and (d) ensuring that the patient understands the diagnostic outcomes and recommendations.

❖ Obtaining Information ❖

The major goal of any encounter is, of course, to obtain information from the patient. For diagnostic testing, this information includes determining the presenting complaint, patient history, and testing outcomes. For audiologic intervention, this information includes understanding the patient's communicative needs and special circumstances.

❖ The "Big" Question ❖

The first and most important question to ask is, "Why is the patient here?" Eliciting the primary complaint allows the clinician to quickly: (a) eliminate any assumptions about the patient's motivations, (b) focus questions and evaluation components on the issue at hand, and (c) guide clinical thinking.

Think of this question as the patient's "story" (Bickley & Szilagyi, 2009). Listening to the patient's story allows the provider to focus assessment on particular areas of concern with an appropriate scope. Use of the patient's own words when possible will help reduce bias in understanding the complaint (Bickley & Szilagyi, 2009). Typically, the most effective way to address this issue is to ask an open-ended question such as, "What brings you in today?" Such a question allows the clinician to most efficiently get to the heart of the problem. Many of the questions a provider would ask about the patient's history will be summarized quickly by the patient following this type of question. Once the patient has answered the question and addressed any other concerns, the clinician can ask more directed questions to further elucidate patient complaints or ask about other potentially relevant areas not addressed by the patient.

Throughout this chapter there are figures that show screen shots of a tablet-based software system, known as eAudio™, used in our clinical practice to document information provided by the patient. Figure 3–1 shows a list of the demographic information that is collected. These screen shots are provided to show visual examples of how such data capture may be organized. It is important to note that the patient's answer to the open-ended question posed previously does not fit neatly into the physical layout of this (or any other) preconstructed list, because patients will have different orders of importance based on their symptoms or concerns. The beginning clinician may struggle somewhat to document the information gleaned from the opening question, and then follow up with closed-ended questions without being redundant and asking the patient the same questions over again. This ability tends to develop with time and experience. Over time, the initial challenge presented by beginning with an open-ended question format will be outweighed by the benefit. Also note that in the figures you will see displayed in this chapter, not all information described in the text is shown in the figure. In the case of our data collection, we have chosen to include an "Add Notes" tab in the left lower corner of each window so that we can capture more specific information

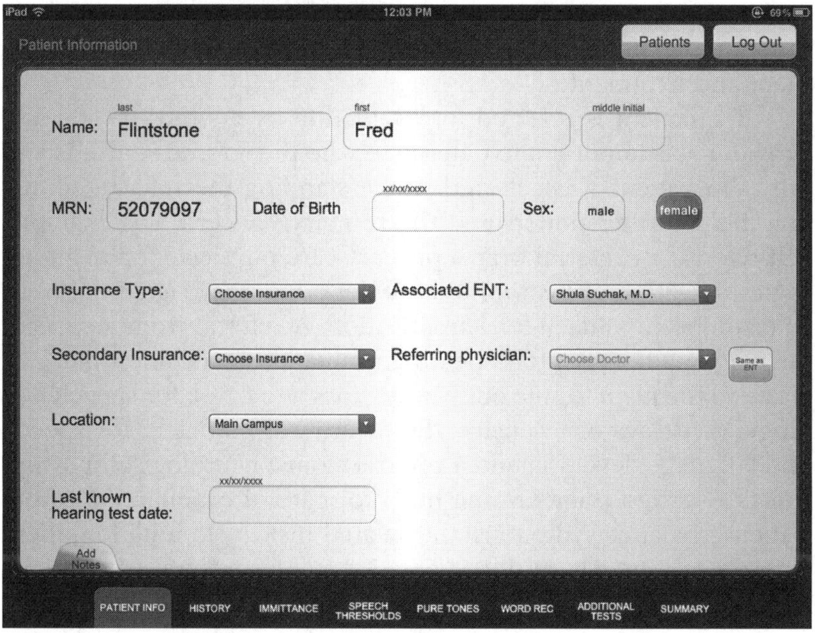

Figure 3–1. Screen shot of eAudio software for demographic information.

that may be provided by a patient. Our strategy is to have a thorough enough information-gathering system to minimize the use of this tab. However, building a system that includes all possible responses from a patient would be too cumbersome to have general clinical applicability. For a number of purposes, including data collection and tracking, we try to avoid the use of prose in "Add Notes" whenever possible.

❖ Referral Source ❖

The source of the referral for audiologic evaluation should be determined during the case history if it is not known prior (see Figure 3–1). Some patients may be self-referred due to perceived problems. In other cases, the patient may be apparently self-referred, but in reality may have come for assessment at the request of others such as family members or friends. Such information will be important in understanding the motivation of the patient to seek assessment and treatment.

If a patient is referred for evaluation by another health care provider, it is important to determine who the referral source is and why the patient was referred. Understanding the referral source may help further understand the primary concern. For example, self-referral, or referral from a primary-care physician for an audiologic evaluation of hearing in an older adult, may signal the need to examine candidacy for amplification. A referral from a speech-language pathologist for a hearing evaluation in a child is likely to relate to the need to rule out hearing loss as a cause for speech and language delays or to ensure that hearing is sufficient for speech and language development. A referral from a neurologist for symptoms of vertigo points to the need for careful examination of the patient's balance symptoms and related history. In addition, there are some cases where documentation of the referral source may be necessary to fulfill requirements for third-party reimbursement for services. For example, the Centers for Medicare and Medicaid Services (CMS) currently stipulates that payment for audiology diagnostic services in the Medicare program can only be made if the test was requested by a medical physician. Documentation of this information is particularly helpful if payment is denied or if records are audited.

❖ The Case History ❖

The ultimate and most important goal of gathering a patient history is to identify important aspects of the patient's medical, social, educational, occupational, recreational, and developmental past that may be relevant to understanding the patient's current and future health. Depending on the specific type of audiologic encounter, goals may be more focused. In the case of a hearing or balance evaluation, all aspects are considered in a comprehensive manner as they could relate to potential hearing or balance problems. In the case of an audiologic treatment encounter, the focus may shift to those aspects of a patient's lifestyle and history that contribute to the potential success for intervention measures. Some case history forms are more comprehensive for obtaining an overview of the patient's general history. Other forms are more focused for specific patient concerns, such as tinnitus or balance, and for specific patient populations, such as children.

Another more pragmatic application of the case history is to document whether the evaluation is being performed for "medical necessity." Medical necessity means that the diagnostic testing is being performed to assist in the diagnosis of pathology by a physician. This information may be important for documentation required by third-party payers for hearing services. For example, CMS requires that audiology diagnostic services be billed to Medicare only if the test is "for the purpose of obtaining information necessary for the physician's diagnostic medical evaluation or to determine the appropriate medical or surgical treatment of a hearing deficit or related medical problem." Appropriate reasons for such tests typically include (CMS, 2012):

- ❖ evaluation of suspected change in hearing, tinnitus, or balance;

- ❖ evaluation of the cause of disorders of hearing, tinnitus, or balance;

- ❖ determination of the effect of medication, surgery, or other treatment;

- ❖ reevaluation to follow changes in hearing, tinnitus, or balance that may be caused by established diagnoses that place the patient at risk for a change in status (e.g., otosclerosis, sudden hearing loss, middle ear disorder);

- ❖ failure of a screening test;

- ❖ diagnostic analysis of cochlear or brainstem implant and programming; and

- ❖ audiology diagnostic tests before and periodically after implantation of auditory prosthetic devices.

The history component of the evaluation can be used to document such information. For example, changes in hearing status would be documented, as would previous diagnosis of hearing- or balance-related disorders. Information pertaining to the symptoms that prompted the physician to order such an evaluation would document medical necessity.

Patient Symptoms and Hearing and Vestibular History

When developing an understanding of patient complaints, information about a particular symptom or problem should be further clarified to assist in diagnosis. Attributes that are particularly relevant to hearing and balance problems include:

❖ location of a particular problem (i.e., left ear, right ear, or both);

❖ severity of the problem;

❖ timing of the problem, including its onset, duration, and frequency of the problem if it is episodic;

❖ factors related to symptom onset, exacerbation of the symptoms, and remission of symptoms; and

❖ symptoms associated with the problem in question (Bickley & Szilagyi, 2009).

Hearing Loss

The patient should be questioned about any current or previous problems with hearing. If the clinician has access to previous audiologic evaluations, they should be reviewed. Note the date of last examination shown in Figure 3–1. If there is a previous hearing evaluation, the patient should be asked whether a change has been perceived since the previous examination. A determination should be made of whether the loss is perceived in the left ear, right ear, or both (Figure 3–2).

The onset of the hearing loss should be determined:

❖ Was the hearing loss congenital or acquired?

❖ If acquired, when did the onset occur with regard to speech and language development?

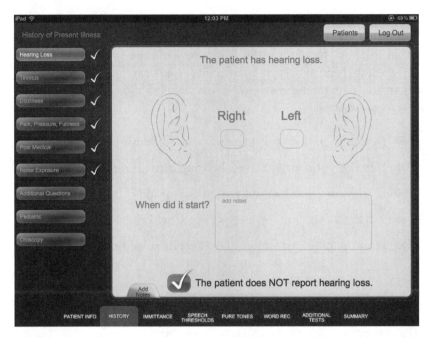

Figure 3–2. Screen shot of eAudio software for information on hearing loss.

❖ Is the loss long-standing?

❖ Did the hearing loss occur gradually over time, or was the onset rapid or sudden?

The patient should also be asked about the stability of hearing:

❖ Does the patient perceive fluctuations in hearing?

The patient should also be questioned regarding the perceived impact of the hearing loss on communication ability:

❖ Does the patient or any family member report difficulty with understanding of speech due to hearing loss?

❖ If so, what situations in particular cause the greatest difficulty?

A hearing handicap inventory, such as the Hearing Handicap Inventory for the Elderly (Ventry & Weinstein, 1982) may be useful in further elucidating the functional impact of hearing loss. If the patient reports hearing difficulty, questions should be asked regarding previous experience with hearing aids and/or assistive listening devices:

❖ Does the patient use hearing aids currently?

❖ Has the patient ever used hearing aids in the past?

❖ If so, how long has the patient worn aids?

❖ What was the patient's experience with hearing aid use?

❖ Is the patient currently interested in amplification?

Tinnitus

The patient's experience with tinnitus should be explored to understand the impact of tinnitus on the patient and to contribute to the diagnostic picture. Tinnitus can be perceived in any number of ways, so it is important to use careful questioning to determine whether the patient experiences sounds or head noises that do not have an external source. If so, the patient should be asked to describe the psychoacoustic qualities of the sound (see Figure 3–3 for example):

❖ Is the sound high- or low-pitched?

❖ Is it like a noise or a tone?

❖ Can the sound be described as anything in particular?

The patient should be questioned regarding whether the tinnitus is perceived only in the left ear, right ear, both ears, or in the head. The onset of the tinnitus should be determined if possible. If the tinnitus fluctuates, it should be determined whether there are any factors that contribute to the onset or changes in tinnitus sensation and whether there are any other symptoms that accompany changes to, or presence of, tinnitus. The ability of the patient

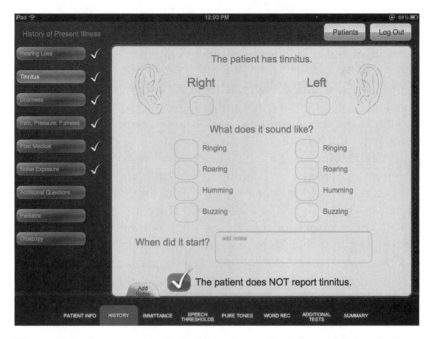

Figure 3–3. Screen shot of eAudio software for information on tinnitus.

to cope with tinnitus should be assessed, and a tinnitus handicap questionnaire, such as the Tinnitus Handicap Inventory (Newman, Jacobson, & Spitzer, 1996) or the Iowa Tinnitus Handicap Questionnaire (Kuk, Tyler, Russell, & Jordan, 1990), may be utilized when the patient complains about tinnitus. The patient's experience with methods of coping with tinnitus should be explored.

Dizziness

For most patients with a presenting complaint of dizziness, the most important aspect of their diagnostic evaluation will be a careful and thorough understanding of their experience with the problem. Patients use a variety of terms to describe dizziness symptoms, any of which may or may not accurately describe their experience. It is important for the patient to elucidate his or her experience with these sensations so that documentation of the symptom can be as accurate as possible to facilitate diagnosis of underlying pathology (see Figure 3–4 for example).

If patients report that they have experienced or are experiencing dizziness, they should be questioned to determine whether the sensation is one of lightheadedness, fainting or near fainting, imbalance, or a spinning sensation, known as vertigo. The patient should be questioned about whether this sensation has led to falls in the past, and if so, these occurrences should be documented. The onset of the symptom should be determined, as well as whether the symptom is episodic or ongoing. If episodic, the typical duration of episodes should be determined. If ongoing, the time since the symptom's onset should be ascertained. The patient should be questioned about associated symptoms such as tinnitus, hearing loss, nausea, vomiting, headache, and pain. The patient should be asked whether any particular events seem to trigger dizziness, including certain positions or movements. Occurrence of other factors that may be associated with dizziness should be documented, including neurologic disease, cardiovascular disease, peripheral vascular dis-

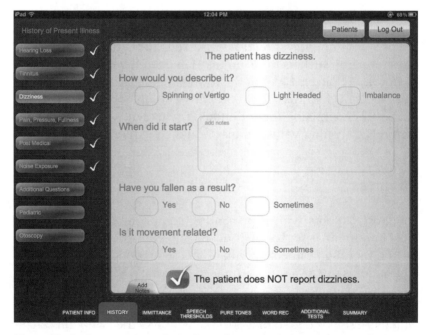

Figure 3–4. Screen shot of eAudio software for information on dizziness.

ease, hyperlipidemia, and psychiatric disease. Use of medications and substances that may cause dizziness should be determined, including alcohol, antianxiety medications, antihistamines, diuretics, antihypertensive medications, antiseizure medications, antidepressants, chemotherapy drugs, antibiotics, and anti-inflammatory medications (Bennett, 2008). The questions should help determine whether recommendations should be made for balance function testing. Assessment of the impact of dizziness on the patient's quality of life through the use of patient self-report measures such as the Dizziness Handicap Inventory (Jacobson & Newman, 1990) may also be a useful determination in some cases.

History of Damaging Noise Exposure

Information of exposure to any potentially damaging noise should be gathered (see Figure 3–5 for example). Typical occupational

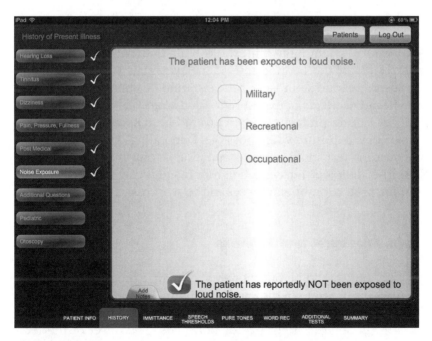

Figure 3–5. Screen shot of eAudio software for information on noise exposure.

noise sources may include military service, factory work, firearms, farm work, and work with loud music or loud machinery. Recreational noise sources often include woodworking tools, firearms, snowmobiles, and cars. However, these are only examples, and patients may underestimate the impact of noise exposure on hearing. Careful questioning in this area is important, and providing examples of common sources of noise to the patient can often assist them in recollecting noise exposure. In addition, many patients assume that reporting past noise exposure is not relevant, so they may need to be prompted to report noise exposure, *even in the past*. If the patient does report exposure to loud noise sources, it should be determined whether the patient uses or used hearing protection when exposed to such noise and whether such protection is or was worn consistently or only occasionally. The frequency and degree to which the individual has been exposed to noise should be ascertained. Are they exposed to this type of noise every day or only very seldom?

In addition, the occurrence of the most recent exposure should be ascertained. If the patient was recently exposed to the noise, such as might occur when a patient is tested following a day of work or recent attendance at a music concert, the patient may experience a temporary threshold shift that will be manifest in the results of the hearing test. If the patient is still experiencing exposure to loud sounds, he or she should be counseled regarding the negative effects of exposure to loud sounds and encouraged to utilize hearing protection when around loud sounds and to minimize noise exposure when possible. Depending on the outcome of the hearing test and possible occupational contributions to hearing loss, the audiologist may need to report significant changes in hearing for protection of employees in the workplace.

Pain, Pressure, and Fullness

The patient should be questioned about any experience with pain, fullness, or pressure in the ears (see Figure 3–6 for example). If any of these symptoms are present, it should be determined whether it is in the left ear, right ear, or both ears. The onset of the feeling should be described and any characteristics of changes in the

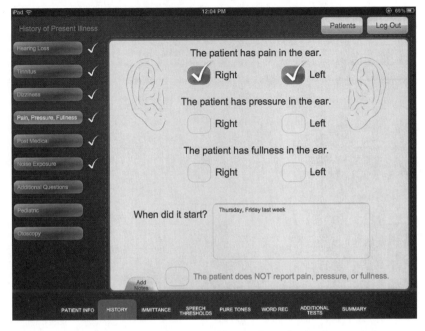

Figure 3–6. Screen shot of eAudio software for information on pain, pressure, or fullness.

sensation should be noted. The patient should be questioned regarding the existence of other symptoms along with any of these sensations.

History of Ear Surgery

The patient should be questioned about any history of previous ear surgeries (see Figure 3–7 for example). Often, patients neglect to volunteer such information under the assumption that if surgery occurred long ago, it is not important to mention. They may also assume that the audiologist has access to information about any surgeries in the medical record. It is important to document in which ear surgery occurred, when surgery occurred, and the type of surgery, if known. In some instances, patients are being seen for audiometric evaluation soon after a surgical procedure.

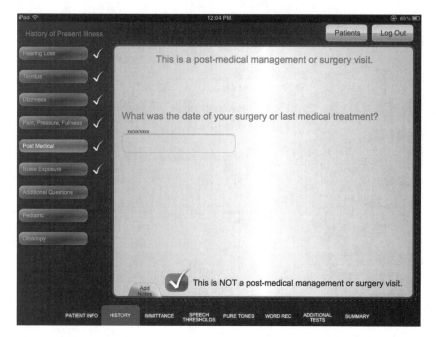

Figure 3–7. Screen shot of eAudio software for information on surgical history.

Certain diagnostic procedures, such as tympanometry and acoustic reflexes, which exert pressure on the tympanic membrane, can cause damage to a recovering ear. In the event that the patient has recently had surgery on the ear, it is recommended that consultation be made with the surgeon to determine whether any diagnostic tests should be avoided.

History of Infections

History of ear infections, otitis media, or otitis externa should be documented. The frequency of episodes should be estimated, especially for younger children. History of tympanic membrane perforations should be reported. The patient should be asked about any myringotomy procedures and/or placement of pressure equalization tubes. The patient should be questioned about drainage from the ear with a description of the color, texture, and frequency of drainage. If previous treatment has been provided, the course of treatment should be understood to determine whether treatment has been completed or it is still under way.

History of Ear Trauma

The patient should be asked about any history of trauma to the ears or ear canal. It should be determined whether the patient has had any force applied to the head that could cause damage to the ear canal or tympanic membrane. In addition, the patient should be asked about the use of cotton swabs or other objects in the ears to determine whether such use may be impacting health of the ear canal.

Use of Medications and Drugs

The patient's use of prescription or over-the-counter medications should be examined. Use of other substances should be assessed as well. Beginning clinicians are often hesitant to inquire about illicit drug use. However, when patients are asked in a matter-of-fact way about drug use, most are surprisingly forthcoming. Certain medications can cause ototoxic and/or vestibulotoxic effects such as hearing loss, tinnitus, and/or dizziness. Some medications cause temporary effects, and others can contribute to these effects permanently. In most cases, greater amount and duration of use contributes to a greater likelihood of potential effects, so the duration of use should be determined as well. Cancer drugs, such as cisplatin, carboplatin, vinca alkaloids, and difluoromethylornithine, can have ototoxic effects. Aminoglycoside antibiotics can have auditory and vestibular toxic effects. Because most patients will not be aware of use of such antibiotics, it is often helpful to ask whether they have ever been treated with an intravenous antibiotic. Most loop diuretics have been shown to cause temporary and permanent hearing loss. Salicylates (aspirin) and nonsteroidal anti-inflammatory drugs (NSAIDs) can cause temporary tinnitus and hearing loss. The malarial drug quinine can produce both ototoxic and vestibulotoxic effects. In addition to these medications, the patient's exposure to industrial chemicals and solvents should be assessed to determine potential hearing and vestibular toxic effects (Campbell, 2007).

If patients report use of medications known to cause temporary hearing loss, such as acetylsalicylic acid (aspirin), they should be questioned about the duration since the last dosage. These medications could create a temporary threshold shift, and knowledge of this possibility will be important in interpreting results and formulating recommendations.

Illnesses and Medical Conditions

Certain illness or medical conditions are known to cause or be associated with hearing loss and/or balance problems. Conductive hearing losses are often caused by otitis media, and a history of ear infections should be elucidated. Viral infections such as mumps and measles are known to cause hearing loss. Meningitis can cause cochlear and/or central auditory hearing loss. Vascular problems, neuropathy due to diabetes, and certain neoplasms are also of concern for hearing loss and balance problems.

Family History of Hearing Loss

The patient should be asked whether there is a known family history of hearing loss (see Figure 3–8 for example). If hearing loss is reported, questioning should attempt to determine whether the family hearing loss has a high likelihood of having etiology that may also contribute to the patient's hearing loss. Information about the onset, degree, and cause, if known, can help shed light on this possibility. The relationship of the family member with hearing loss to the patient should be ascertained.

Gathering Information About Children

The evaluation of children requires attention to a host of other areas of concern that are particularly relevant to understanding the cause of hearing loss and how it may impact the child's overall development. When evaluating children, among the most impor-

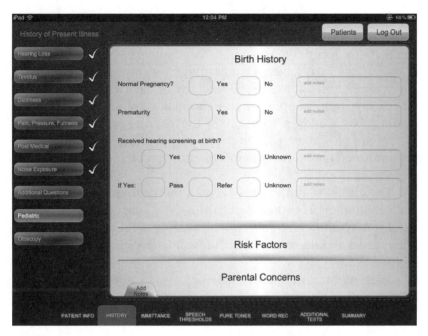

Figure 3–8. Screen shot of eAudio software for information on birth history.

tant questions to be asked of the caregiver is whether there are concerns regarding hearing. In addition, when assessing children, family history of hearing loss takes on even greater importance.

For children, caregivers should be questioned about pregnancy, birth, and postnatal history. Any problems or concern during the pregnancy should be noted (see Figure 3–8 for example). Maternal illnesses such as cytomegalovirus (CMV), herpes, rubella, syphilis, and toxoplasmosis during pregnancy can cause hearing loss and should be noted (for a summary of auditory disorders in infants, see Stach & Ramachandran, 2008). Any genetic testing outcomes or suspicion of neurofibromatosis, osteopetrosis, Usher syndrome, Waardenburg, Alport, Pendred, Jervell and Lange-Nielson, Friedreich ataxia, and Charcot-Marie-Tooth syndrome should also be noted. Information regarding use of medications or substances during pregnancy should be gathered. Common concerns during the time surrounding birth and immediately after are hypoxia, hyperbilirubinemia, particularly at a level requiring transfusion, use of extracorporeal membrane oxygenation (ECMO), use of ototoxic medications, length of stay in a neonatal intensive care unit (NICU) of more than 5 days, head trauma, and chemotherapy. Infants who have craniofacial anomalies, particularly of the ear or ear canal, ear pits or tags, and temporal bone anomalies are at higher risk for hearing loss. Children with any of the previously mentioned risk factors are at higher risk for developing hearing loss and should be monitored over time (Joint Committee on Infant Hearing, 2007) (see Figure 3–9 for examples).

For children and infants seen in the postnatal period, information should be gathered regarding the outcome of newborn hearing screening and subsequent hearing screenings. History of otitis media should be explored, including frequency and duration of episodes.

It is important to assess whether overall development of the child is within normal limits or whether there is a possible global

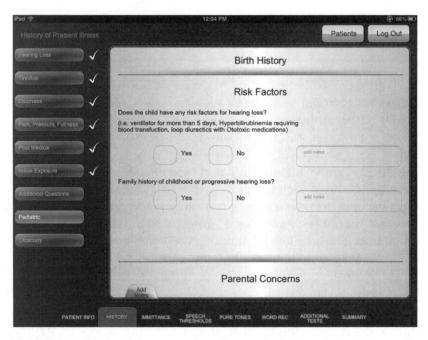

Figure 3–9. Screen shot of eAudio software for information on infant risk factors for hearing loss.

developmental delay. Such delays have the potential to impact speech and language development, and the developmental level of the child will be important in selecting appropriate evaluation techniques. Lags in physical development may be clues for potential vestibular problems in very young children.

Caregivers should be questioned about speech and language development (see Figure 3–10 for example). Specific questions regarding age-appropriate milestones for speech and language development should be used to screen for potential problems. For example, does a 2-year-old child put two words together? For preschool and school-age children, information regarding special services the child is receiving should be gathered, such as speech-language pathology, psychology, physical therapy, or occupational therapy services, or any other services the child may be receiving in school. The parent should be asked about the child's school performance and whether there are any concerns regarding hearing in the classroom.

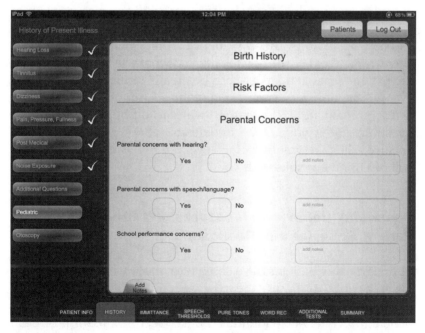

Figure 3–10. Screen shot of eAudio software for information on parental concerns for hearing loss.

❖ Setting Expectations for Testing Procedures ❖

During the initial stages of the appointment, the goals of the encounter should be addressed. The patient is expected to provide appropriate information and to behave in certain ways during the encounter. By explaining the goals for the session to the patient, the provider will help the patient focus efforts toward achieving those goals. In addition, the patient will likely appreciate the respect that is conveyed by being asked to actively participate in the care encounter.

The audiologist should also explain to the patient exactly what will happen during the appointment. Providing the patient an idea of the time that will be required for any procedure is helpful in beginning to set expectations for the appointment. The patient should also be informed of the actions that will be taken during the visit to help structure the appointment and address any potential barriers to successfully completing the necessary tasks. In diagnostic encounters, the use of appropriate instructions and setting expectations will allow the audiologist to obtain behavioral and objective test results in an effective and patient-sensitive manner. Many patients have never participated in an audiologic evaluation and may be anxious. By providing clear information to the patient about what to expect during testing and what will be required from the patient, fears and anxiety can be greatly reduced. For example, "We will be doing a test to check your hearing today. The testing takes approximately 30 minutes. I will start off by asking you some questions about yourself to understand about your hearing and balance. Then we will be doing several different tests. Afterward I will discuss the results with you."

Describing Behavioral Measures and Expectations for Patient Behavior and Responses

Although many patients have some idea about what to expect during behavioral testing of hearing, specific tasks required of the patient will need to be made explicit prior to testing. For many people, previous behavioral testing has been in the form of hearing screening. In this case, patients are not listening for the softest sounds they can hear, but rather a suprathreshold signal in most cases. Therefore, during threshold testing the patient must be made aware to respond to sound every time it is heard, even if the sound can just barely be heard. The type of response desired by the audiologist will also need to be explained. Many patients will have an assumption about the type of response they should make, such as hand-raising, and they will utilize this response unless instructed differently. Most patients will be unfamiliar with the techniques of bone-conduction testing and masking. It is important to explain to patients what they can expect to hear and what the desired response should be. In terms of describing masking, it is often helpful to introduce the masking noise to patients after the explanation so that they can understand which sound they should ignore. When changing tasks, the patient should be alerted to the new task and provided with appropriate instructions. For patients with poor speech understanding, it may be necessary to remove earphones and speak directly to the patient face-to-face so that the patient may utilize visual cues.

Some sample instructional wording is described in the following for various tasks:

- ❖ Speech-recognition threshold:
  I am going to put some earphones into your ears now. I am going to say some words to you, and I would like you to repeat the words back to me when you hear them . . . even if they are very soft and hard to hear, just take your best guess as to what the word might be.

- ❖ Pure-tone air-conduction:
  Now you are going to hear some tones. I would like you to say "yes," every time you hear the tone. Even if the tone is very faint, say "yes."

- ❖ Word recognition testing:
  You are going to hear a man's recorded voice asking you to say some words. I would like you to repeat back the word that he tells you to say.

- ❖ Pure-tone bone-conduction with masking:
  I am going to put a device behind your ear to present more tones. I would like you to say "yes" every time you hear the tone. Even if the tone is very faint, say "yes" no matter which ear you hear the tone in. Some of the time you may hear some wind noise in your other ear. If you hear the wind noise, just ignore it, but tell me "yes" every time you hear the tone.

Describing Electroacoustic and Electrophysiologic Measures and Expectations for Patient Behavior

Although patients often have an intuitive understanding about how behavioral pure-tone testing proceeds, they are often intrigued and/or confused about how objective measures contribute to the overall picture of hearing function. When using measures such as immittance audiometry, otoacoustic emissions, and auditory-evoked potentials, it is helpful to patients and family members for the audiologist to provide a succinct, yet accurate description of what is occurring.

❖ Immittance measurement:
  I am going to put this soft earphone in your ear and you will hear a sound and feel some pressure changes. You will also be hearing some loud sounds in both ears that we use to measure a reflex in your ear. We are doing this to see how well sound travels through your ear canal and ear drum.

❖ Otoacoustic emissions:
  I am going to put this soft earphone in your ear and you will hear some sounds. The sounds are transmitting to what is called your "inner ear." In the inner ear, there exists what are called "hair cells" that move in response to the incoming sound. The movement of the hair cells actually creates a sound wave as well. That sound travels back out through the ear system to the ear canal where a microphone records the sound. When we're able to record that sound, it tells us that the inner ear is functioning the way that it is supposed to.

❖ Auditory-evoked potentials:
  I am going to be pasting electrodes on your scalp and putting earphones in year ears. You will be hearing some loud clicking sounds. Your job is to close your eyes and be still. Falling asleep is allowed and encouraged. We are doing this test to see how well the nerves of hearing are functioning.

CHAPTER 4

Audiologist as Counselor: Telling the Story Well

When considering the various ways that ideas can be communicated, perhaps the most useful principle is to tell the story well. It is common in everyday life to communicate all manner of information, stories, and questions. In the real world, most people are adept at tailoring their intended message to their audience, using appropriate terminology and conveying information in a way that the receiver will understand. When people tell stories to their friends, they structure the stories to make them concise while conveying all of the information necessary for understanding. They use language and terminology that the listeners can understand. They use appropriate affect and timing, and they highlight the most important points of the stories in a variety of ways. Communicating with patients is similar, except that the story is told within a clinical context and with a professional tone. Thinking about how most appropriately to tell the story will likely convey the message well.

In the interest of telling this story well and not cluttering the discussion, we will primarily limit our examples to the audiologic hearing evaluation, because this is the most common diagnostic experience for patients and audiologists. However, you should consider how these principles can be applied to any other facet of audiologic evaluation or treatment.

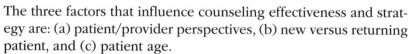

❖ **Factors That Influence the Conversation** ❖

The three factors that influence counseling effectiveness and strategy are: (a) patient/provider perspectives, (b) new versus returning patient, and (c) patient age.

Your patients' perspectives are necessarily different from yours as a provider. The patient may be familiar with audiometric testing results or may be completely unfamiliar with them. Patients may know what caused their hearing losses or be very worried about the cause. They may wear hearing aids or want to avoid doing so. Parents may have other children with hearing loss or may never have thought about childhood hearing loss and its impact on speech and language development. An individual patient's perspective will necessarily vary depending on experience.

In contrast to the patient's unique perspective, your perspective on the patient's hearing loss will not be unique. You may be seeing the tenth patient today with bilateral moderate sensorineural hearing loss or the third baby today with transient conductive hearing loss. One of the most challenging aspects of informational counseling of patients is remembering that this is each patient's only hearing loss. One of the most important challenges you face is avoiding treating patients as audiograms rather than as individuals with communication needs. Your effectiveness in counseling depends on your ability to perceive the uniqueness of each encounter.

One of the most important factors influencing counseling strategy is simply whether the patient is a new or returning patient. The seasoned patient will require little explanation about the hearing testing results and their impact. First-time patients are likely to be considerably more anxious about the nature of their problems and the potential solutions. You may need to spend considerably more time on content counseling and on emotional counseling with the latter group.

One other factor that will influence the strategy for counseling will be the age of the patients. Adult patients will want to know about the cause of their hearing problems, whether their general health is at risk, and whether the problem is medically treatable. They will be aware of the problem they are having and will generally be willing participants in the discussion. Parents of infants and children identified with hearing loss require what can sometimes be a considerably different approach to the discussion. This will vary as a function of age of identification of the loss, whether the parent suspected a problem, and so on.

These various patient factors combine, then, to make each encounter different. Although it is sometimes difficult to know what your individual patient's perspective might be, there are some commonalities that should help guide you.

❖ Emphasizing the Important ❖

Once the history has been gathered, clinical testing performed, and impressions formed, it is time to talk with the patient or family about the outcomes of testing. In all forms of communication, the most effective way to accomplish communication goals is to focus on what is actually important and to find a way to emphasize this during communication, whether in verbal or written form. Once the goals for a particular encounter are determined, a few vital outcomes need to be conveyed to patients:

❖ What do we know?

❖ What don't we know?

❖ What next?

❖ Explaining It ❖

One of the most challenging aspects of communicating with patients is describing what was learned in the encounter. This element of communication can be difficult due to the sophisticated nature of auditory and vestibular system structure and function and the technical management strategies often used by audiologists. Patients will have varying knowledge of these systems, and it is necessary to explain outcomes in a simple but comprehensive and useful manner. However, understanding the questions that are of greatest importance to the patient can help guide your strategies for communicating this information.

When considering how to talk with a patient or family about diagnostic results, it is important to consider their perspective in the interaction. Potential barriers to communication should be identified and dealt with when possible. The specific concerns of patients will differ depending on the type of encounter and the patient's personal experience with hearing health care. Some patients have never had an audiologic evaluation, and others may have been receiving hearing care treatment for years. For auditory diagnostic testing, most patients are typically interested in understanding several major issues. Patients often want to know:

- ❖ "Is there anything wrong with me medically?"

- ❖ "Do I have hearing loss?" "How bad is it?"

- ❖ "Do the results you obtained make sense for the problems that I'm having?"

It is important for the audiologist to develop strategies for conveying the answers to these questions in clear and understandable terms.

Terminology

In the quest to make information about hearing loss, tinnitus, and other complex phenomena understandable to patients or their families, language and terminology are often used that are different than that learned in the classroom or used with other professionals. Whereas the goal of making these concepts more understandable is correct and important, use of terminology that is inaccurate or inconsistent can actually be more confusing to a patient. It is of great benefit to a patient if the correct terminology is used when explaining hearing and hearing loss. Many patients will be evaluated by a physician subsequent to diagnosis of hearing loss, and it is helpful to the patient when consistent terminology is used among providers to describe the hearing loss. Furthermore, many patients will seek information from outside sources, such as the Internet, to help understand their hearing loss. If a patient has hearing loss, the terms "conductive" or "sensorineural" should be used to inform the patient of the loss.

Although it is important to use accurate terminology when talking with patients, clarity is an important consideration as well. In order to help patients understand their hearing loss, the use of more readily understood terminology, if accurate, should be used. For example, when describing the acoustic characteristics of hearing loss, it may be helpful to describe the psychological correlates of the physical properties of acoustic events. For example, most patients are familiar with the concepts of *loudness* and *pitch*, whereas *intensity* and *frequency* are likely to be more difficult to comprehend.

There will, of course, be some patients who are familiar with these concepts. For example, other health care professionals, engineers, and musicians typically understand terminology that others might not. This familiarity is typically discovered quickly through interaction with the patient, and it can be helpful to such patients to explain outcomes using more technical language. However, even with much knowledge there may still be terms and concepts that are unfamiliar to such patients, and the audiologist should be vigilant to guard against assuming too much preexisting knowledge.

When Less Is More

It is often tempting to include all the information gathered during an evaluation in the explanation to patients and other providers. Providers often feel as if giving more information to patients will help them better understand hearing loss. However, brevity is also an important factor in allowing patients to understand hearing loss. Most patients are likely to be overwhelmed by excessive amounts of information. Retention of information and depth of understanding is likely to be greatest when the most important information is presented clearly and is uncluttered by superfluous facts. The most useful communication will focus on answering those concerns that are the major goals of the encounter.

In some cases, using visual information, such as a diagram of the ear and analogies to other more commonly encountered problems, can be helpful when discussing function. For example, describing how conductive hearing loss makes sound quieter and showing a diagram of where the conductive loss occurs in the ear is often helpful for patients to understand what is happening.

Some clinicians routinely utilize the audiogram itself to describe hearing loss to the patient. If this is used, it will be necessary to orient the listener to the graph before proceeding. This would include explaining what is characterized on each axis and what the symbols on the graph refer to. Using the audiogram can be of benefit in some cases. For example, using a chart of familiar speech sounds superimposed on the patient's audiogram can help the patient understand what speech sounds are being missed in conversational speech. This may give the patient greater insight into why he or she can "hear" speech, but not "understand" it.

On the other hand, orienting a naïve listener to the audiogram can be an intensive effort and may ultimately not achieve the desired effect of education. Consider how long it took for you as a clinician to learn to read and interpret an audiogram effectively. You probably did not fully understand the concepts upon your introduction. Yet, for patients who are having their first audiologic evaluation, we are asking them to learn and understand information about the audiogram, apply this knowledge to understand their hearing loss, and then make decisions about how they would like to proceed as far as treatment. This is a lot to ask. Several years ago, our clinic used a computer-based audiometer system on a trial basis that temporarily made it difficult for us to have a physical copy of the audiogram as we counseled the patient. We had to learn to use our words and simply talk to the patient about our findings. To our surprise, in most cases we found this strategy far more effective for counseling than having the audiogram to talk about. We were much more able to focus on the primary concerns of the patient and were more "in tune" with questions that the patient had. In general, we came to view the audiogram as an obstacle to counseling, rather than as a helpful tool. It was a relief not to be burdened by describing information about the test itself, which is really what the audiogram shows, but rather to focus on the hearing function and its impact on the patient. We did not, however, find that this was the case for every single patient. Some can and do benefit from examining the audiogram. It is up to the audiologist to evaluate each patient as an individual to determine the best means of conveying information, rather than using the same approach for everyone.

Nature and Degree of Hearing Loss

For patients who have hearing loss, the next step is to help them understand the nature and degree of hearing loss. When discussing the type of hearing loss, it is important to use consistent and correct terminology to describe the loss. Use of lay terms such as "nerve deafness" are often confusing to the patient, particularly when the loss is later discussed with other health care providers or when the patient seeks outside information about the loss. The terms *sensorineural* or *conductive* should be used as appropriate. When mixed hearing loss is present, it is helpful to describe each type of hearing loss distinctly. Often a diagram is helpful in illustrating to the patient where the sensorineural or conductive components to a hearing loss can occur. In many cases, the patient will ask whether the hearing loss can be medically treated. In most cases of sensorineural loss, of course, the hearing loss is permanent, and the patient should be informed of this. Questions regarding medical treatment of conductive or sensorineural hearing loss should be directed to the referring physician.

The degree of hearing loss should also be explained to the patient. Again, consistent use of terminology is helpful, and terminology such as mild, moderate, moderately severe, severe, and profound are readily understood by most patients. When the degree of loss differs as a function of frequency, it is often helpful to describe the degree for "low-pitch" and "high-pitch" sounds. It is important to be accurate in describing hearing loss to a patient, but also to provide simple, easily understood information. Patients who have had prior hearing tests may wish to know whether their hearing has changed since their previous evaluation. This information should be provided to the patient as well.

Impact of the Hearing Loss on Communication

Another goal of the encounter is to help patients understand the congruence between the hearing loss and the communication problems they are experiencing. For patients who are likely to understand it, use of diagrams showing speech sounds on the audiogram with the patient's thresholds overlaid may be a helpful tool for counseling the patient regarding sounds that are audible and those that are not. This information can be conveyed verbally as well.

For example, for patients with sloping hearing loss, describing how they are missing many consonants, which are high pitch, and hearing many vowels, which are low pitch, explains why they can hear that someone is talking but cannot understand what they are saying. Use of word recognition scores can also be helpful in counseling patients about how they are able to perceive speech in quiet once it is made loud enough to hear. It is particularly important at this stage to provide an empathetic ear as patients describe their particular communication challenges resulting from hearing loss and to provide acknowledgment of the congruence between test outcomes and perceptions. Overall, the audiologist should help patients understand how the hearing loss is contributing to particular problems they may be experiencing.

Recommendations for Additional Health Care Management

If there is information that was not attainable during the evaluation, for whatever reason, it is important to emphasize to the patient or family what is and is not known. This is important for helping the patient or family understand the need for follow-up and putting the information presented into context.

Patients may question the audiologist regarding the cause of their hearing loss. In the majority of cases, the cause of hearing loss cannot be determined definitively, and the audiologist must take care not to assign the cause of hearing loss to a particular illness or event. The diagnosis of medical pathology lies with the referring physician. For patients who have such questions, referral should be made to the referring physician to provide such answers. However, it can be explained to the patient that there are numerous causes for hearing loss. If the patient questions whether noise exposure or aging can cause hearing loss, these factors can be affirmed as potential causes of hearing loss when appropriate.

Recommendations for Audiologic Management

The terminology used and complexity of audiologic recommendations can be challenging to the goal of providing clear and comprehensible information to a patient. Again, the specific concerns of the patient will differ depending on the type of clinical encounter and the patient's experience with hearing health care. Once questions have been answered regarding the patient's hearing, patients typically want to know:

❖ "Can my hearing loss be fixed or cured?"

❖ "If not, what are my options?"

❖ "What do *you* think I should do?"

❖ "What do I do next?"

The audiologist must be able to provide answers to these questions in a manner that allows patients to understand the ramifications of management issues so that they can make appropriate decisions.

Candidacy for audiologic treatment is often an important question for most patients. Generally, patients are looking for the audiologist's assessment of whether they "need" hearing aids or some other form of intervention. It is important for the audiologist to provide professional judgment regarding the need for amplification based on both audiologic outcomes and assessment of the patient's communication issues and needs. It is also helpful to provide a general understanding of prognosis for benefit from hearing aids. Although the clinician cannot judge conclusively the patient's potential outcomes from hearing aid use, the patient should be counseled regarding appropriate expectations. A patient with moderate hearing loss and good suprathreshold hearing is likely to benefit considerably from modern hearing aids. In contrast, a patient with poor word recognition will need to have expectations guided accordingly.

A final major goal of the interaction is to ensure that the patient understands the next steps to be taken. If a physician referral is recommended, the patient should be provided with information for scheduling, and any paperwork that the patient needs should be provided. Any follow-up needed for audiologic intervention should be discussed, and patients should have a clear understanding of what they need to do after they leave the office.

Patient Perspective: Adults

As stated at the beginning of this chapter, when considering how to talk with a patient or family regarding hearing loss, it is vital to remember that the patient is likely to have a different perspective than the provider. As an audiologist, hearing loss is encountered on a daily basis. There is nothing novel about it. For a patient or family member, hearing loss is often a new experience about which almost nothing may be known. In addition, many patients and families have little to no understanding of the potential impact of hearing loss, particularly when hearing loss is of a degree that is sufficient to impact speech perception, but less severe than "deafness." The fact that patients often have little to no previous experience with hearing loss means that they must be offered a great deal of empathy and education.

It is important to remember the role of the audiologist in relation to the patient. The patient and family are the experts on the functional consequences of the patient's hearing loss. They live with the hearing loss and the communication consequences daily. The audiologist is the professional who is trained to diagnose and quantify the hearing loss, to educate the patient and family on the hearing loss, and to provide recommendations for intervention when appropriate. It is necessary for the audiologist to simultaneously acknowledge the role of the patients as expert on their experience with hearing loss and provide the information and recommendations that patients need in order to make decisions regarding what to do about it.

The provider's primary goals in talking with patients tend to be related to conveying appropriate and useful information. This is typically referred to as "content counseling." It must be understood, however, that many, if not most, patients will have some type of emotional reaction to discussion of hearing loss. Remember that each patient is different, with different circumstances and history that create a unique background into which hearing loss is incorporated. The importance of empathy on the part of the audiologist cannot be overemphasized.

The diagnosis of hearing loss may be an emotional experience for patients and families. Many patients believe that their own hearing loss is a sign of "getting old." They may be uncomfortable accepting a condition that they stigmatize or associate with something contrary to their own self-identification. Other patients may express relief at knowing that, although they have hearing loss and other symptoms such as tinnitus, this is not a sign of medical illness or cognitive impairment. The clinician should be prepared for a host of possible emotional expressions.

In addition to the impact of hearing loss itself, many patients have emotional contexts associated with acquisition of the hearing loss. One author recalls during experiences in a Veterans Administration hospital that when discussing hearing loss several patients reported that they remember the exact moment when hearing was compromised during battle. These patients relived the moments when a blast injury occurred or during episodes of extended noise exposure from repeated use of firearms in combat. Patients told their stories about seeing fellow soldiers and friends dying in the battlefield when hearing loss was incurred. These stories were accompanied by emotional responses, such as crying, even though the incidents occurred decades previously. It is also not uncommon to find that patients present for hearing evaluation following the illness or death of their spouse. Often, the experience of dealing with a host of unfamiliar individuals with a vital need for effective communication in such situations highlights to patients how poor their communication ability has become and how much they may have relied on a spouse to act as a buffer against confronting these communication challenges in the past. In some cases, the patients become emotional in relating their present circumstances, and they may associate the loss of hearing with grieving for a loved one.

Patients themselves may find that the diagnosis of hearing loss adds to the grief that they may experience about the knowledge of their own mortality. In some cases, hearing loss accompanies potentially fatal illness or disease in patients. A clinician may see patients who are undergoing chemotherapy treatments or who have chronic disease processes. They may see patients who are extremely elderly and who report that they feel they will not live much longer. It is important to recognize the patient and his or her affective state and to provide an empathetic attitude in which patients are able to tell their story. Many patients may view the audiologist as an important individual to whom they can talk about the emotional or life impact of their hearing loss. They expect the clinician to have an understanding of the impact of hearing loss that will allow the clinician to empathize with their situation.

Newer clinicians will spend much time mastering the ability to provide content counseling to patients in an effective and useful manner. As the clinician becomes comfortable in this role, he or she will have the opportunity to tune into the affective responses of patients during these encounters.

Patient Perspective: Children

Imagine being a parent of an infant brought in for hearing assessment. The first question is whether the child has hearing loss or
not. If so, how much and what does it mean for the child in terms
of his or her future? And once there has been time to process the
news—"What do I do next?"—rest assured that unless the parent asks about how these conclusions were reached, the process
in reaching them is unimportant. The child and the conclusions
reached regarding that child's hearing are the focus of the parents'
concerns. So the audiologist should start there. There is no need to
burden the anxious parent with details about the process used to
reach the conclusions. This is why it is often a good strategy, when
communicating with patients and other providers, to begin with the
conclusions. The discussion should start with the communication
of conclusions and recommendations. Discussion can then proceed, if necessary, with the play-by-play of the methods used and
the specific results obtained.

In some cases, audiologists are taught during training to report
their findings by beginning with the process, followed by the outcomes. In a training situation, it is extremely important to educators
that students demonstrate their understanding of the process and
their ability to perform the process competently. When in training,
it is necessary to justify outcomes by demonstrating that the student performed the assessment accurately and, furthermore, that
the appropriate conclusions were reached. However, in practice,
patients and providers will take it for granted that practitioners are
competent in their skills. It will not be necessary to communicate
in great detail the process of getting to the conclusions reached.
It may also seem natural to begin with the history, followed by
results, followed by conclusions, simply because this is how the
process is performed clinically. However, in considering the next
step, communication, the strategy for how results are communicated should now have its own important place in the process.
There are important outcomes to communicate, and one important
way to emphasize them is to get the order right.

Although many of the perspectives described previously apply
to the diagnosis of hearing loss in children, parents and caregivers
may have different or additional emotional responses and immedi-
ate concerns. Just as with adults who have hearing loss, parents are

typically unaware of the particulars of hearing loss and its impact on communication. Audiologists know, however, that the impact of hearing loss on children can have different sequela than hearing loss that develops in adults. Parents may need to be educated about the likely impact of hearing loss on speech and language development and oriented to the need for intervention.

The emotional consequences of a diagnosis of hearing loss can be significant. When infants are diagnosed with significant hearing loss, the parents may well progress through a process of grieving regarding hearing loss similar to the stages of grief associated with death and dying (Kübler-Ross, 1969). Stages include: denial, anger, bargaining, depression, and acceptance. These "stages" may occur and reoccur at any point as the individual with hearing loss and family members adjust to hearing loss throughout the lifespan. The audiologist, in dealing with the hearing loss, will often be the person on the receiving end of the emotional responses that accompany these stages. An example, provided by Clark and English (2004), is when a patient or family member who is dealing with feelings of anger surrounding a hearing loss lashes out at the audiologist. Realizing that this response may stem from feelings of grief should help minimize the negative impact of the reaction on the clinician. It is important to allow the family to experience and deal with these grief experiences rather than attempt to minimize, hurry, or detract from them. As parents progress through the stages of grief the audiologist must provide appropriate empathy, education, and recommendations.

For parents who receive an initial diagnosis of hearing loss in an infant or child, the experience can be devastating, with untold emotional consequences. Parents may cry or appear numb, or they may even appear engaged and motivated to aggressively pursue intervention. The emotional reaction of parents is often influenced by the timing of identifying the hearing loss. Parents of a child who has had a progressive hearing loss or who was identified "late" are often already aware of the hearing loss from having observed their child's development, and they are just awaiting confirmation from the audiologist. There may be little denial, but the parent may feel substantial guilt over the time lost before identification occurred. Parents of an infant diagnosed with hearing loss, particularly with no known risk factors, are often in denial regarding the hearing loss. They have not yet witnessed the developmental impact of the hearing loss and may not be willing to accept the audiologist's input as to the potential consequences of untreated hearing loss. Such parents may be angry at the audiologist for being the messenger of this information.

Holland (2007) discusses common parental concerns when faced with a disability. These relate to others' acceptance of the child, the safety of the child, the child's ability to function independently, and the happiness of the child. Financial and other logistical concerns about extra time needed to parent a child with hearing loss can also be present. When applied to issues such as utilizing hearing aids or cochlear implants, these acceptance and financial issues can become important to parents. Most patients, and especially parents, want to know what caused the hearing loss. They may have concerns about their other children or about family planning issues. They may have concerns about other potential problems associated with the hearing loss. They may fear what hearing loss will mean for the child's future.

Patients and parents of children who are diagnosed with hearing loss typically experience shock that compromises their ability to understand and retain new information. Although it is important to provide information, it should not be unexpected when this information is not remembered. Despite our best efforts, patients may have difficulty understanding or remembering information presented to them. It is often effective to have patients explain their diagnosis, recommendations made, and instructions for follow-up, back to the provider—a process known as "teach back"—to ensure that there have been no misunderstandings or that important information has not been overlooked. It may also be helpful to provide supplementary written materials to which patients may later refer if information is forgotten.

For parents who are confronted with a diagnosis of hearing loss in a child a myriad of other concerns may be manifest.

Clinical Notes: Managing "Functional" Patients

Some patients exaggerate or feign hearing loss. The rationale for such behavior can be extremely varied, but the goals for the audiologist remain the same—to identify the patient behavior and then to obtain information that is as accurate as possible regarding hearing status. Although it can be a frustrating experience to be faced with exaggerated and feigned hearing loss in a patient, it is not advantageous for the audiologist to allow such feelings to interfere with interaction with the patient. Often, the most useful technique for eliciting appropriate patient responses is to reinstruct the patient regarding expected behaviors during testing. In some cases, the patient may not actually understand the behavioral testing paradigm. In other cases, the patient is willfully exaggerating the loss and such reinstruction can provide the patient with an opportunity to "save face" by blaming inconsistencies on lack of understanding of the task. In such cases, the patient is alerted to the fact that the audiologist is aware that behavioral results are not accurate, and the patient has the opportunity to provide correct behavioral responses without having to admit to exaggeration or feigning. Beyond these measures, if patients continue with invalid responses, in most practice settings the best suggestion is to have patients schedule an appointment for objective prediction of hearing sensitivity by auditory-evoked potentials.

PART II

Written Communication with Health Care Providers

CHAPTER 5

Written Communication

At some point in the evaluation and treatment process it will be necessary to put your actions, findings, and thoughts into written format. The written documentation and reporting of audiologic encounters may be in many forms, including medical record documents and reports, letters to a referral source, and progress notes. The nature of what you write within these documents may also vary as a function of the referral source or intended reader. This chapter summarizes the importance of knowing with whom you are communicating and the various types of reports that may be written.

❖ Knowing with Whom You Are Communicating ❖

The information learned from the audiologic assessment is often used by other health care providers for various purposes. In these cases, it is important to understand what the other health care provider's questions will be. For example, if a child is referred for hearing testing prior to a speech–language evaluation, the most likely question of interest to the provider is, "Does the child have a hearing loss that is interfering with speech and language development?" In this case, the most meaningful information that the audiologist can provide is, "Hearing is sufficient (or insufficient) for normal speech and language development."

Audiologists often work closely with otolaryngologists who use audiologic information to help medically diagnose specific pathologies of the auditory system and formulate medical treatment decisions. Some of the most common questions of interest to otolaryngology providers that can be gleaned from the audiologic evaluation include:

- ❖ "Is there dysfunction of the auditory system?"

- ❖ "If yes, where in the system does disorder exist (outer/middle ear, inner ear, and/or retrocochlear)?"

- ❖ "Can the hearing disorder be treated medically?"

- ❖ "Is the hearing loss causing a communication problem for the patient?"

- ❖ "If the hearing loss cannot be treated medically, what are the recommendations for management of the hearing loss?"

When describing information learned and recommendations, it is important to recognize the diversity of familiarity and experience that various health care providers will have with assessment outcomes. Otolaryngology providers will have depth of knowledge regarding diagnostic and treatment options for hearing disorders. Primary-care and other specialist providers typically will bring less knowledge to the table. Just as with conveying information to patients, it is important to match your explanations to the knowledge base and experience of the receiver.

The variety of roles of other health care providers who might be interested in audiologic evaluation outcomes requires that we also tailor our communication to match the perspective of the provider. Many different types of providers refer patients for audiologic evaluations. Primary-care physicians, emergency department physicians, pediatricians, neurologists, speech–language pathologists, and otolaryngologists are typical sources of referrals in most settings. These providers all differ in their level of expertise in diagnosing and treating disorders of the auditory and vestibular systems. For example, generalist physicians and pediatricians typically want to know whether they can treat the patient themselves or whether the patient requires referral to a specialist or surgeon. These physicians also need to understand the importance of audiologic screenings for infants and children. Neurology providers typically are interested in differentiating between peripheral and central sites of pathology and whether the patient needs to be referred to another provider for assessment and treatment. Speech–language pathologists may recommend audiologic evaluation to rule out hearing loss as a contributing factor to speech and language disorder and whether hearing loss is sufficient for typical speech and language development.

Otolaryngologists and otologists can be assumed to have a greater depth of knowledge of the workings of the ear. Typically, they want to know if there is something they can do to remediate the hearing loss through medical treatment. In other cases, they may wish to document hearing status as an adjunct to necessary medical treatment. These physicians are concerned with the potential for retrocochlear disorder. They are concerned about the outcomes of vestibular or balance evaluation. Otolaryngologists and generalist physicians need to understand audiologic interventions and prognosis to provide medical clearance for hearing aid use. Otologists need to understand audiologic candidacy for cochlear implantation and outcome prognosis for this treatment. These physicians rely heavily on audiologic evaluation outcomes in diagnosis and treatment strategies. They will require less is terms of providing general information about audiologic dysfunction and require more targeted and sophisticated information to assist in the diagnostic process and treatment planning.

❖ The Challenge of the Electronic Medical Record ❖

When determining how to communicate with the many providers who may need to understand audiologic evaluation and intervention outcomes, it is important to keep the needs and perspectives of that provider in mind when planning your communication strategy.

A challenge to this customization occurs when written reports are included in an electronic medical record. In some institutions, the electronic medical record (EMR) or electronic health record (EHR) provides a historical record that may be easily accessed by a variety of provider types. The challenge here is to convey appropriate information to the referral source and to provide information that can be both sufficiently detailed for providers who understand much about auditory function and audiologic evaluation, but easy enough to be understood by providers who understand little. The report must essentially be all things to all potential readers. In this case, an easily understood summary, followed by more detailed interpretation and documentation, will best serve the long-term interests of all parties.

❖ Reporting Versus Documentation ❖

Among the many written documents that health care providers generate are those that provide documentation and those that serve as reports. In considering how to write your findings for any evaluation or patient encounter, it is important to differentiate between documentation and reporting. Documentation refers to the recording of results of testing and details of patient encounters in the medical record. Reporting, on the other hand, refers to the summarization and interpretation of evaluation findings and patient encounters. An example common to audiometric evaluation would be establishing hearing thresholds for a patient. The documentation in this case would be the actual audiogram and individual thresholds. The report would consist of an interpretation of those documented findings, for example, calling the loss a high-frequency sensorineural loss.

❖ Types of Records ❖

Medical Records

The medical record refers to the systematic documentation of a person's medical history and care. It is the summation of all documents related to the patient's medical care. The medical record may be kept in a paper format, electronic format, or combination of these. It consists of a variety of information, including identifying information, health history, examination and evaluation findings, test results, prescriptions, referrals, educational materials provided, instructions for follow-up care, and, in some cases, billing information.

Letters

Letters provide information about a patient's evaluation and care to an outside referral source. Letters can be sent electronically, or hard copies can be generated. Letters are similar to medical reports in that the information about the patient is summarized and interpreted. If documentation is included, this is generally an attachment to the letter. The letter is addressed to a particular individual and is written to address the concerns of the letter recipient. A copy of the letter becomes part of the permanent medical record.

Progress Notes

Progress notes document and report on periodic and continuing encounters with patients. Typically, when patients are undergoing audiologic intervention services with an audiologist, they are seen numerous times. Whether patients are using hearing instruments, cochlear implants, or other implantable systems, or undergoing audiologic rehabilitation, progress toward better hearing and communication is the long-term goal. In most cases this goal is not realized immediately, regardless of the technological sophistication of the instrumentation. As patients are seen for regularly scheduled or as-needed follow-up, progress notes serve to document and report the encounters.

The goals of writing progress notes are to document the encounter, record updated information regarding the patient's hearing health care status, and report on the plan for progress toward better communication for the patient. The progress note contains information such as why the patient was seen for the appointment, what was accomplished during the session, and the plan for the future.

For example: "*Mr. Jones was seen today for a scheduled hearing aid check appointment. The patient reported that his right hearing aid was 'not working.' Inspection of the hearing aid revealed that the receiver was clogged with cerumen. The hearing aid was cleaned and a listening check revealed good sound quality. Electroacoustic analysis revealed that the hearing aid was functioning according to specifications. Real-ear measures demonstrated that the hearing aid was functioning as expected. The patient was satisfied with the performance of the aid following cleaning and reported relief at having*

*his hearing aid working. Cleaning and maintenance of the hearing
instrument was reviewed with the patient. Mr. Jones will return for
his six-month follow-up appointment in June or sooner if needed."*

Encounter Notes

Every contact with a patient should be documented. If the patient
was seen by the audiologist, it was for a reason, no matter how
small. The information exchanged between the audiologist and
the patient should be captured and available to facilitate communication with other providers. Encounter notes can be used to
document communications that occur between the audiologist, or
his or her office staff, and the patient. The contact may occur in
many ways: telephone, E-mail, in person. Regardless of the method
of communication, documentation of the information shared will
allow the audiologist to recall important information at a later time
or will allow another professional to understand the clinical situation in the absence of that audiologist.

Supplemental Materials

Supplemental materials are additional, usually written, materials
that help patients recall information presented in face-to-face ses-
sions and that provide additional, more in-depth information about
particular topics. These materials are often used to expand on topics discussed with patients. Supplemental materials should be written in easy to understand style and in language used by laypeople.
The font should be large enough for patients who may have visual
difficulties. Contact information should be included for patients in
case they need clarification of the information on the materials.
Translated materials should be available for patients who have
limited English proficiency.

Medical–Legal Evaluation

Whereas most types of written reports focus on clinical care of
patients, a medical–legal report provides professional judgments

regarding the diagnosis and probable cause of hearing loss. When providing such information, documentation of evidence to support impressions and recommendations is of vital importance to the reader. The audiologic component of such an evaluation should contain a statement of the validity of the hearing evaluation, the type and calibration status of the equipment utilized to gather data, the occurrence of prior noise exposure to determine potential for temporary threshold shift, and a statement of hearing handicap. See Dobie (2002) for discussion of calculation of hearing handicap and further information on medical–legal evaluation.

CHAPTER 6

Documenting

Dr. Lawrence Weed gave a grand rounds presentation to a group of medical professionals in Chicago in 1971. During this lecture, Dr. Weed equated medical records to patients themselves. He pointed out that there is no way a provider can retain in his or her memory every detail of a patient's history, symptoms, diagnoses, or treatment plans. The only way to have access to such information is to write it down. If the patients were present, this information could be asked, assuming that they could remember every aspect of their own medical history, which is unlikely. In the absence of the patient, the medical record *is* the patient. It is the compilation of all information about the patient that the provider can access. In addition, if another provider were to assume care of the patient, that new provider must have access to sufficient information to continue to treat the patient. In the absence of written documentation, the other provider would have no means to understand the history of the patient's treatment and the particulars of what the patient may need. The importance of the medical record in the care of the patient cannot be understated. We will get back to Dr. Weed and his important thoughts in Chapter 7 when we discuss reporting.

To be effective the medical record must be organized so that the provider can understand what it contains. A disorganized medical record presents obstacles to effective patient care. The information must be accurate and, above all, it must facilitate communication.

The audiologist contributes to the patient's medical record, whether this is within his or her own practice or within a larger medical setting. Furthermore, the audiologist should be cognizant that no matter where the record is originally maintained, if the patient changes providers, the record may end up in another facility's medical record system. Thus, the audiologist should always assume that the record may be accessed at some point by another provider and care should be taken to record information so that it can be communicated effectively.

❖ Documenting ❖

In health care settings it is important to document data and findings so that they can be accessed in the future as needed. In Chapter 5, we made a distinction between documenting and reporting. An understanding of that difference helps in guiding how and what kind of information is maintained in the medical record. Recall that *documentation* refers to the recording in the medical record of results of testing and details of patient encounters. In contrast, *reporting* refers to the summarization and interpretation of the testing and encounter.

Documenting outcomes and how they were obtained is important for a variety of reasons. These include demonstrating the process for reimbursement, having a record from which to understand the process in the future as may be needed for continuous follow-up for the patient, and a host of other possibilities. The seasoned clinician understands that the medical record generated during an audiology encounter will be viewed again. The range of reasons that it will be viewed again is broad; from a referral source viewing the record, to the audiologist viewing the record prior to reevaluation, to a Medicare audit, to medical–legal review in deposition. Understanding that the record will be seen again is compelling enough reason to be thorough, accurate, and organized in the documentation of a patient encounter.

❖ The Electronic Medical Record ❖

With increasing frequency, health care providers are using electronic formats for archiving medical records. The electronic medical record (EMR) or electronic health record (EHR) provides a mechanism by which obtained information can be stored and accessed. The use of electronic medical records provides enormous power and flexibility to the clinician to easily locate documentation and reports for a particular patient. When numerous physicians and providers have access to a patient's medical record, the provider has a powerful tool by which information can be garnered about the reason for referral of a patient and any relevant patient history. The ability to obtain information in this manner has the potential to enhance patient care and bring greater efficiency and effectiveness. The EMR provides a means by which patients can have greater continuity of care among providers.

For all of the benefits and advantages associated with electronic medical records, implementation can create challenges. In any EMR system, information is available from providers who have little to no relationship to the patient's audiologic needs. There is risk for a professional to venture into areas of the patient's medical record that would reasonably be considered "none of the audiologist's business." It is important when accessing patient records that the ease with which this may be accomplished not lead the provider to attempt to access information that is not immediately relevant to the patient's hearing or balance health history or to the presenting complaint.

Another challenge that clinicians must be cognizant of is the tendency to replicate information from previous medical records without verifying the accuracy of the information with the patient. In some cases, previously recorded medical history may, in fact, be inaccurate. Replicating such information without verification will perpetuate inaccurate information throughout the patient's medical record and has the potential to result in inappropriate diagnostic indicators and/or intervention recommendations. In addition, previously recorded patient information may have changed in the time between prior contact with the patient and the current encounter. It is important that the clinician not accept as "truth" the information contained in the medical record and that information is verified with the patient.

❖ The Data: Making It Clear and Getting It All ❖

In Chapter 7, we review the evidence base and advantages of what is known as "itemized" reporting. This type of strategy, essentially a checklist of findings, is ideal for recording the data captured during the audiologic evaluation. By using an itemized format, readers of the document can locate and use information reliably and efficiently, because it is presented in the same place and manner each time. Another benefit of the itemized format is the checklist-like nature provides a means to ensure that all necessary data are collected appropriately. Formatting the data in a manner that emphasizes particular findings can be an important contribution to creating a record that easily communicates information to the reader. More is said about this in the section on the audiogram later in the chapter.

❖ Documenting the Hearing Evaluation ❖

The data gleaned from the audiologic evaluation should be included as documentation in the patient's record, following the assessment and plan components of a report. The case history serves as the "subjective" component of the record. The "objective" component includes the otoscopic examination, immittance results, threshold testing results, speech audiometry results, and otoacoustic emissions results.

Case History

When reporting the case history, any current or past symptoms or history relating to hearing or balance issues should be reported. Typically, this section is also the area in which the presenting concern of the patient is identified. This section of the written report should ideally be an itemized list of answers to the questions asked at the beginning of the patient's evaluation. An in-depth description of this information can be found in Chapter 3.

In reporting on the information gleaned from a case history, some information elicited will be relevant to the patient and some will not. For example, from a small sampling of information, a given patient may report hearing loss bilaterally and a history of noise exposure, but not tinnitus, vertigo, or ear pain. In order to minimize the confusion of another provider hearing or reading a report regarding this patient, it is helpful to focus your communication on those characteristics that pertain to that particular patient. There are several ways to do this. One is to report only those present-ing symptoms and avoid reporting any problems a patient does **not** have. In this case, the reader of such a report would need to assume that you had assessed the unreported information during your evaluation. However, research shows that physicians often do not make that assumption. Rather, they assume that, if the test was not mentioned, it was not completed (Bosmans, Weyler, De Schepper, & Parizel, 2011). An alternative strategy is to highlight abnormal results in some way. For example, formatting can be used to bold, highlight, color, or capitalize a letter of abnormal findings so that attention is drawn to them visually. In this way, the reader is not forced to sort through history to determine what is charac-teristic of this patient and what is not.

Otoscopic Examination

Reporting on the results of the otoscopic examination should high-light any abnormalities that may indicate the need for referral or that may interfere with auditory function. Such reporting should involve a description of the observed phenomenon and avoid ter-minology that is diagnostic in nature. Some examples include:

❖ Normal otoscopic examination;

❖ Normal otoscopic examination: presence of in situ tympa-nostomy tube;

❖ Abnormal otoscopic examination: presence of occluding cerumen;

❖ Abnormal otoscopic examination: presence of foreign object;

❖ Abnormal otoscopic examination: unknown debris or other substance in the ear canal;

❖ Abnormal otoscopic examination: drainage in the ear canal;

❖ Abnormal otoscopic examination: bulging/red tympanic membrane;

❖ Abnormal otoscopic examination: apparent tympanic mem-brane perforation.

Immittance Results

Immittance results should be recorded in the documentation section.

Typical data to include:

❖ equivalent ear canal volume;

❖ tympanometric peak pressure;

❖ tympanometric width/gradient;

❖ static immittance;

❖ acoustic reflex thresholds (ipsilateral and contralateral);

❖ acoustic reflex decay, presence or absence.

To further facilitate communication, clinicians may find it helpful to characterize tympanometry outcomes by the Jerger classification system (Jerger, 1970). This classification system is familiar to many types of providers and may be more meaningful when utilized. This system includes:

❖ Type A (normal);

❖ Type As (decreased static immittance);

❖ Type Ad (increased static immittance);

❖ Type B (flat);

❖ Type C (significantly negative tympanometric peak pressure).

Also, many providers have sufficient familiarity to glean substantial information from a physical rendering of the tympanogram. Inclusion of the picture, where able, can be helpful.

Hearing Sensitivity

Hearing sensitivity results are interpreted for the reader in the report section of the document. The audiogram then provides the raw data that support the interpretation.

The audiogram is a fundamental component of the documentation process. Although it can take various forms, it is often included in the medical record as the actual graph of hearing sensitivity as a function of frequency. Because of its ubiquitous use in audiology, it is worth reviewing its history to understand both its usefulness in documenting outcomes and its challenges to the documentation process.

A History of the Audiogram: A Picture Worth a Thousand Words

The audiogram was first developed by Fletcher and Wegel and described in a publication by Fowler in 1930. Harvey Fletcher and R. L. Wegel were hearing scientists, and Sir Edmund Prince Fowler was an otolaryngologist. Where was the input from audiologists who were using the audiogram to convey clinical findings? Well, of course there were no audiologists yet. The "father of audiology," C. C. Bunch, published the book *Clinical Audiometry* in 1943, by which time the earliest conventions for conveying hearing sensitivity were well entrenched. Audiometry was initially performed by technicians, who turned their results in to the physician for interpretation. In this case it was necessary to have a system for conveying not only the audiometric thresholds but also the methods used to determine the thresholds. These included the ear tested, transducer type, and whether masking was used. In a 1951 publication, Fowler further described his rationale for the symbols chosen to populate the audiogram, including the concept of "straightening out" the line for normal hearing sensitivity and plotting the graph in a downward direction. He felt that these conventions " . . . provided a chart that the clinician could visualize better."

Considerable changes have occurred to the audiogram since its inception. In particular, decibels hearing level (dB HL) is used instead of sensation units as the measure for intensity. The symbols used to plot hearing sensitivity also evolved over time. In 1974 the American Speech-Language-Hearing Association (ASHA) provided guidelines for the use of audiogram symbols. Interestingly, some conventions adopted by these guidelines were used despite previously raised objections to the potential difficulty of deciphering symbols on the audiogram, such as using the "X" and circle symbols together, which could obscure visualization of either (Fowler, 1951).

Jerger (1976) followed ASHA's recommendations with another set of symbols, proposed for use in scholarly publications, which minimized the number of symbols used and plotted ear-specific data on separate graphs. Despite contrasts with the ASHA symbol set in which ease of interpretation was illustrated, these recommendations were not widely adopted for clinical use. Currently, the American National Standards Institute (2004) and ASHA (1990) guidelines for audiometric reporting are similar and are the most widely used methods for graphically reporting audiometric data. No evidence base known to the authors currently exists for valuing any one method of reporting over another for use in effectively communicating audiometric findings.

In the ASHA (1990) and ANSI (2004) systems, there are different symbols for each ear, for each manner of sound transduction (air conduction or bone conduction), and for indicating whether the nontest ear was masked or unmasked.

❖ A circle (○) is used for the right ear unmasked air-conduction threshold, and a triangle (△) is used for the right ear masked air-conduction threshold.

❖ A "less than" sign (<) is used for a right unmasked bone-conduction threshold, and a left square bracket ([) is used for right masked bone-conduction thresholds.

❖ An "X" is used for the left ear unmasked air-conduction threshold, and a square (□) is used for the left ear masked air-conduction threshold.

❖ A "greater than" sign (>) is used for left unmasked bone-conduction thresholds, and a right square bracket (]) is used for left masked bone-conduction thresholds.

❖ Additional, less standardized symbols may be used for sound field testing (S or W), indicating nonspecific ear for bone-conduction thresholds (^ or □) and so on.

❖ To indicate "no response," when the patient does not respond behaviorally to stimuli at equipment limits, an angled arrow is typically added to the symbol, with the arrow pointing toward the left (225° angle) for right-ear symbols, and toward the right (135° angle) for left-ear symbols.

Symbols may be plotted for both ears on the same audiogram, or the ears can be separated onto two different graphs. Traditionally, blue ink was used to plot left ear symbols and red ink was used to plot right ear symbols to further differentiate ears that are plotted on the same audiogram. This convention has generally fallen by the wayside over the years, as duplication of audiograms by photocopying, scanning, and faxing is done in black and white, thereby eliminating this additional information.

In the Jerger (1976) method, the ears are always separated, so there is no need to utilize different symbols for different ears. A circle is used for air-conduction thresholds and a square is used for bone-conduction thresholds. These same two symbols are then left unfilled to indicate that no masking was used for the non-test ear, or shaded to indicate that masking was used. This results in a total of four symbols: unmasked air-conduction, "○," masked air-conduction, "●," unmasked bone-conduction, "□," and masked bone-conduction, "■." In this system, symbols are not plotted when there is no response at equipment limits.

Most clinics tend to utilize the ANSI (2004) or ASHA (1990) symbols. However, there are differences in the conventions used within clinics. Whereas the unmasked air-conduction symbols are often constant among clinics, there is less consistency with regard to the symbols used for other threshold measures. Because there are numerous possibilities for plotting thresholds on the audiogram, the use of a key is necessary to avoid confusion on the part of the reader.

Some clinics prefer not to use an audiogram, instead utilizing a table in which audiometric thresholds are recorded. This method is commonly used in the Veterans Administration Medical Centers and other medical centers that use electronic medical records systems extensively. The audiogram itself does not lend to seamless integration to an electronic system at this time, so a tabular format for recording audiologic data is highly useful in this situation.

It should be noted that the authors strongly believe that technology available for recording and obtaining results should not dictate how the results are communicated if the system does not make sense for your purposes. This issue becomes important because there is increasing pressure to utilize computer-based systems for reporting audiologic information. It is imperative that the solution chosen actually works for your clinical situation.

When the actual audiogram is used in the medical record, there are numerous variables to consider in choosing the recording method. One is whether ears should be separated or combined. The preference of the authors is to separate ears onto different graphs to eliminate the symbol overlap that often occurs

---

The "Science" Behind the Audiogram

Of historical note, Fowler (1951) also recommended the following:

❖ The right ear should be represented by a dot (·) and the left ear by a circle (○). The reasons for this were that the symbols could be overlapped without creating visual distortion (the dot inside the circle). He also suggested that "both the dot and the circle represent openings, in this case the external auditory canals" and that "these symbols are easy to remember," whereas "other symbols are wholly arbitrary and do not bring before the mind any suggestive resemblance or association with the things they represent." He also felt that these symbols were advantageous because "dot" suggests dextra and "circle," phonetically at least, suggests sinistra.

❖ Regarding colors, Fowler suggested " . . . red (suggesting right) should be used for the right ear and some other color, say lemon or lead (suggesting left), for the left ear. Blue also may be used appropriately for the left ear, since the word blue prominently contains the letter "l," suggesting left."

We cannot help but wonder if the reader of such an audiogram might not confuse lemon with yellow or lead with gray, thereby obscuring interpretation. But perhaps because yellow prominently contains the letter "l," it is fine.

when ears are combined. In addition, by reducing the number of symbols included on one graph, air–bone gaps are more easily visualized. The downside, according to some, is that it may be more difficult to detect bone-conduction asymmetries when the ears are separated.

Another issue of importance is the recording of "no response" symbols. In our experience, "no response" symbols are often mis-read when the audiogram is visualized. This leads to the impression of hearing being present, when the exact opposite information is attempting to be conveyed. It may be more beneficial to simply write NR for "no response," to leave the symbols out altogether with the assumption that the reader of the test will trust that you completed your evaluation appropriately, or to write on the audiogram that "no responses were obtained to masked bone-conduction at x Hz at equipment limits."

Despite the chaos suggested by the previous depiction, the audiogram is a useful method for simultaneously documenting degree, configuration, type, and symmetry of hearing sensitivity.

Speech Audiometry Results

Documenting speech audiometric results is fairly straightforward. For speech thresholds, documentation should include the threshold levels obtained as well as the type of stimuli presented (e.g., spondees, digits) and the response required from the patient (e.g., speech awareness, speech recognition). For word recognition testing, documentation should include the percentage correct score, the presentation level of testing, the word list(s) utilized, and the method of presentation (recorded vs. live voice). The latter information is particularly important when considering diagnosis of retrocochlear dysfunction or comparing test results over a period of time. In addition, presentation level is important in interpreting speech audiometry results. If the presentation level is not of sufficient intensity, word recognition performance will be compromised. The clinician who uses these data for comparative purposes must understand at what intensity level speech was presented.

The Use of MLV

The use of monitored-live-voice (MLV) testing has consistently resulted in inconsistent scores when used for retesting and has been shown to have artificially high scores when compared to the use of recorded materials (Roeser & Clark, 2008). As such, word recognition scores obtained with MLV cannot be used for valid assessment of retrocochlear dysfunction, nor can they be a valid indicator of changes in performance over time. If MLV is used for word recognition, it is of utmost importance that the clinician referencing the data has access to information on how the materials were presented.

Otoacoustic Emissions Results

Typically, when otoacoustic emissions testing is utilized during a hearing evaluation, it is as a cross-check of behavioral measures. An interpretation should be made of whether otoacoustic emissions (OAE) results validate behavioral measures. Examples of descriptions are: "Distortion product (or transient, depending on the method used) otoacoustic emissions consistent with normal cochlear outer haircell function"; "Distortion product otoacoustic emissions consistent with pure-tone results"; and "Absence of distortion product otoacoustic emissions consistent with middle ear dysfunction."

Functional Hearing Loss

In the case of suspected functional hearing loss, the final version of the hearing test results should reflect only the results deemed to be accurate. Documentation of results believed to be inaccurate serves only to create further confusion in future evaluations. Although the audiologist may use a "worksheet" audiogram at the onset, the final version of the audiogram, which will become a part of the patient's permanent medical record, should reflect only those results the audiologist believes to be accurate. If the patient's behavioral responses are deemed to be inaccurate, a statement relating this is the only information that should be included on the pure-tone audiogram, although objective measures may be included.

In some practice settings it is mandated that the audiologist include threshold measures for patients, even when they are suspected of having functional hearing loss. In such a case, a note should be made of the impression that "audiometric threshold measures are likely suprathreshold."

When attempting to describe the results of the evaluation, comments can be made about consistency of results. When cross-check measures suggest a potential functional hearing loss, the phrase "consistent results could not be obtained" may be used, or "behavioral measures are inconsistent with objective measures" when this is the case. Such information, as well as the lack of responses plotted on the audiogram, will alert the reader to the inconsistency of results during testing and the possibility of functional hearing loss.

Reporting Reliability

The aforementioned treatment of invalid or inaccurate behavioral responses can be used to eliminate the need to report reliability of results, at least when testing adult patients. In some cases, these patients are merely unable to comply with testing procedures, and the suprathreshold nature of responses should be described.

Unfortunately, the terms typically used to describe reliability of results lack any functional definition when applied to audiologic evaluation. Even when reliability is judged to be less than ideal, there is no agreed upon terminology for defining reliability, and the interpretation of the meaning may suffer. If reliability is judged to be "fair," does this mean that the patient is uncooperative, sleepy, did not understand the directions, is cognitively impaired, is malingering, or something else? Use of a reliability rating for adults lacks sufficient usefulness to be included in most reports.

One case in which reliability may be useful is in the case of testing children. In adult testing, of course, the assumption is that when adults are capable of being tested with conventional measures, they are capable of appropriately responding to stimuli. Use of one term to describe less than ideal reliability is simply not enough information for any clinician to make appropriate use of the evaluation results. For children, however, there are often periods of development when it is not uncommon for testing outcomes to be less than ideal. Or, in some cases, children are distracted for any number of commonplace reasons. In these cases, a measure of reliability can be useful to a clinician who may evaluate the child in the future. If reliability is less than ideal, information should be documented about the testing paradigm and the child's behavior. Such information should be helpful in tailoring future evaluations to obtain valid responses.

CHAPTER 7

Reporting:
Telling the Story Well

One of the most important aspects in the provision of health care is reporting results of an evaluation or treatment outcome. The challenge of reporting is describing what was found or what was done in a clear, concise, and consistent manner. The nature of a report can vary greatly, depending on the nature of the medical record, the setting, and the referral source to whom a report is most often written.

Throughout this book, we have tried to stress the importance of distinguishing between documentation and reporting of test results. As you learned in the previous chapter, *documentation* is the preservation of examination and test results in a medical record. *Reporting* is the summary of that documentation. As an example, when you carry out immittance testing, you will obtain a large amount of detailed information about the tympanogram, static immittance, reflex thresholds, and so forth. That is important information to document as part of the patient record. However, what you write in your report might be "normal middle ear function," an important and clear summary statement about these test results.

Documenting audiometric data is crucial, but most readers will not understand what all of it means. So it becomes incumbent on the audiologist to summarize these data for reporting purposes. In some form or another, all of these documented data are interpreted and converted into report form as a means of effectively communicating the findings. It is not uncommon in reporting to fail to compartmentalize these two issues.

One of the simplest ways to communicate effectively is to delineate and separate those aspects of the report that serve as documentation from those intended to summarize the outcome. The reader may understand the detail, but it is unlikely. Although thoroughness is an important attribute of documentation, succinctness is an important attribute of reporting.

In many clinics reporting is done in a summary section on the audiogram form. In other clinics, a separate document is generated, usually intended for the referral source or third party. Regardless of the form of reporting, there are some fundamental rules for generating effective results. One is to organize the report in an order that makes sense. Another is to use clear, concise, consistent terminology.

❖ Getting the Order Right ❖

Many health care reporting strategies use a traditional organization, from an elaborate description of the history, through the assessment of methods, and on to results and recommendations. We have found, however, that in a busy health care setting, that sequence is nearly the reverse of what is important in terms of the effectiveness of reporting. More modern approaches, designed to facilitate efficient communication of the finding, place the interpretation of findings ahead of the documentation of test results. For an electronic record, where the report and documentation may be combined, it may be useful to sequence the results so that the conclusions come first and the documentation last. This way, anyone reading the report will be able to get to the conclusions without having to wade through the details.

The History of SOAP Notes

A commonly used structure for audiologic and most other medical reporting is the SOAP note format. SOAP is an acronym that stands for "subjective," "objective," "assessment," and "plan." This acronym is routinely used by health care professionals to organize both their thinking about a patient's situation and to record this information in a logical manner.

- ❖ The "**S**ubjective" component refers to the patient's report of symptoms and problems.

- ❖ The "**O**bjective" component refers to the information collected by the medical professional, including physical examination and other evaluations (e.g., the results of an audiologic evaluation as shown on the audiogram).

- ❖ The "**A**ssessment" component refers to the clinician's determination of function or disorder that is explained by the aforementioned data.

- ❖ The "**P**lan" component refers to the recommendations for treatment or intervention, if any.

SOAP notes are currently typically used to structure the record of clinical encounters with patients. This is interesting when considering the origin of the SOAP note. SOAP notes were originally devised for medical reporting by Dr. Lawrence Weed, who was introduced in the previous chapter. In his 1968 work on "Medical Records that Guide and Teach," and in a grand rounds session video recorded in 1971, Dr. Weed suggested that a patient's medical record should be "problem oriented" rather than "source oriented." By this he meant that the medical record should be structured to focus on the particular issues that a patient was having, rather than organized according to the contacts or encounters that a patient had with the provider. It was noted that, in examining a patient's medical chart, there was no narrative describing the patient's overall experience. He suggested that the chart should include an ever-updating "problem list." The problem list would be a "table of contents" to the remainder of the record that documented each encounter, examination, and progress note in detail. The problem list would provide an overview of the patient's problems. The SOAP format was originally designed to expand the "problem list" with a simple list of vital information regarding the problem and what was being done about it.

For example, if a patient presented with the problem of "hearing loss," this would be included in the patient's medical record on the problem list. This may be one of many patient problems that include diabetes, vision loss, etc. If a patient presents to the physician with the problem of "hearing loss," the medical record may include statements like the following in the list:

Problem List

1. Hearing loss

    S: Difficulty hearing, left ear. Ringing sound, left ear. Fullness, left ear.

    O: Normal otoscopic examination and pneumatic otoscopy.

    A: Rule out sensorineural hearing loss.

    P: Refer for audiologic evaluation.

In the original SOAP note, in the case where a patient is seeing some form of specialist, such as an audiologist, the patient has already been essentially "filtered" regarding the "problem." Presumably the problem is already "hearing" or "balance" in nature. The audiologist would then "update" the "problem list" by confirming and/or refining the subjective experience of the patient, providing new objective information, providing a new assessment of hearing or balance status, and a new plan for treatment, if any.

This "problem-oriented" model for medical records was never embraced fully by the medical profession. More than 40 years later, most medical records continue to be organized in a source-oriented, rather than problem-oriented manner. The SOAP note itself, though, was widely adopted. It was recognized that structuring the patient encounter in this manner was helpful to those professionals who were learning to communicate with patients and to organize their thinking regarding medical treatment. Use of the SOAP note has evolved, so that now, in our widely used method of audiologic reporting, and throughout the health care community, the SOAP note has become a means of structuring patient "encounters" rather than supporting a "problem" list. That is, for each visit that the provider has with a patient, a record is created that is outlined according to the subjective experience of the patient, the objective data gathered by the provider, the assessment generated by the provider, and the plan for treatment or follow-up generated by the provider.

A Communication Problem

For the audiologist at least, this format may present a problem for communicating effectively among providers. In our institution, the SOAP note format for reporting audiologic results has been used historically. In order to understand how well we were communicating with our referring physician providers, we conducted a retrospective study in which we reviewed 6,000 audiologic reports and compared them to the physicians' reports (Ramachandran et al., 2011). In almost all cases, the physicians describe the audiologic findings as part of their report. Essentially, the audiologic findings became part of the "O" or "objective" component of the physician's record. Results showed that there was an incongruence in explaining audiologic findings in about 25% of the cases. It was clear that there was room for improvement for communication among providers.

Why is the SOAP note not ideal? Consider the consumer of this form of report from the perspective of a problem-oriented medical record. What information is the consumer of the information (i.e., the referring provider) likely to require from the specialist? Is it a review of the clinician's experience with the patient, or is it information necessary to update their "problem list?"

We surveyed our readily available otolaryngology colleagues to ascertain the answer to this question. These physician providers frequently need to call upon other providers such as radiologists, pathologists, oncologists, psychologists, audiologists, speech-language pathologists, and so on, to provide valuable diagnostic information that they then use to develop a diagnosis and treatment plan for their patients. In many cases, more than one piece of additional information is required for each patient. These providers estimate that they receive over 100 reports per day from other laboratories and specialists. Because these otolaryngology providers are specialists themselves, their patients were referred to them by some form of primary care provider, who must also sort through all of these reports. Clearly, these providers need to contend with an enormous amount of information. Other strategies are emerging to provide a better method of communicating important information to the provider.

The APSO Note

One solution to the challenges described previously is to structure the reports in such a way to emphasize the important outcomes first. The "assessment" and "plan" components of the SOAP note are of greatest relevance to the referral source. The "subjective" and "objective" components are important and necessary to document, but if the referral sources were experts in obtaining and interpreting such results, they would not have requested a referral to begin with. It is the assessment and plan of the specialist that is of greatest interest to the referring source and, as such, the report should be structured to most effectively and efficiently communicate the desired information.

Rather than a SOAP note format, an APSO note format may be of greatest utility, where the "assessment" and "plan" come first, and "subjective" and "objective" data come later. In focusing on the goals for communication, it is important to remember that patients and other providers are most interested in the outcomes. The process may be unimportant to them. Patients and other providers seek our services because they have concerns about hearing and/or balance. Typically, their concern will focus simply on the answer to the question, "Is there a hearing and/or balance problem?" And if there is a problem, they will want to know a few other specific things about it. How you came to the conclusion that there is a problem is generally at the bottom of the list of their concerns.

An APSO note based on the aforementioned information might include:

A: Right ear: Normal middle ear function and moderate sensorineural hearing loss.

Left ear: Normal middle ear function and mild sloping to severe sensorineural hearing loss.

P: Binaural hearing aid amplification.

The S and O would follow with the documentation recorded by the audiologist.

❖ Critical Thinking ❖

Instructors have emphasized the use of SOAP notes for years as a useful tool for training student clinicians. What makes the SOAP or APSO note so attractive to instructors? The logic inherent in the process is the key. The clinician must first gather data about the patients and their situations to formulate an assessment and plan. Therefore anything stated in the assessment and plan should have clear links to the data component of the record. For example, if the assessment includes a statement about abnormal middle ear function, the objective data contained in the documentation section should support this impression. As another example, if a component of the audiologist's plan is to recommend balance function testing, the subjective data contained in the documentation section should support the patient's experiences with the need for the evaluation (i.e., patient complaints of dizziness that suggests a vestibular cause). The information found within the data provides justification for the assessment and plan components. Likewise, the assessment and plan components address the patient concerns and objective findings discovered via the audiologic evaluation.

❖ Templates and Checklists ❖

The level of structure within a report can vary considerably. On one end of the continuum is free-text or prose, where there is little or no structure. Next is a semistructured report. SOAP or APSO notes would be an example of this. Further along the continuum is a template format or structured report that is more detailed and standardized than the traditional SOAP note. At the other end of the continuum is what is known as an "itemized" report, which is a standardized list of findings and interpretations, much like a checklist.

Templates and itemized reports, the most detailed options, have been used in other specialties of health care, including radiology and pathology. These specialties fulfill a consultative role for referring physicians, which is often the role that the diagnostic audiologist fills as well. Evidence from these specialties has shown that the format of reporting information has important implications for communication, for thoroughness in patient history-taking and examination, and for helping to guide the thinking of providers. When examining physician perceptions of how they prefer to receive or write reports, both referring physicians and radiologists reported that they preferred itemized reports over prose (Bosmans et al., 2011; Grieve, Plumb, & Khan, 2010; Naik, Hanbridge, & Wilson, 2001). When asking radiologists and referring physicians to report on content and clarity, Schwartz and colleagues (2011) found that itemized reports were rated higher than prose reports in both. Pathologists, who have published association guidelines on what should be included in reports, rated itemized reports as higher in completeness according to those guidelines (Idowu, Bekeris, Raab, Ruby, & Nakhleh, 2010; Messenger, McLeod, & Kirsch, 2011). The study by Messenger and colleagues (2011) found that nonspecialist pathologists did not report as many incidents of samples that cause concern for pathology compared to specialist pathologists when using prose for reporting. However, when the nonspecialist pathologists used an itemized format for reporting, their reports were more complete, and they also identified the same rates of suspect samples as the specialist pathologists. It appears that the reporting methodology created a means for structuring the thinking and interpretation of the provider, which resulted in improved outcomes as well as better reports.

❖ Emphasizing the Important and Drawing Attention to the Abnormal ❖

Providers report that they prefer having detailed reports and want "pertinent negatives" included in the documentation (Bosmans et al., 2011; Naik et al., 2001). This means that if there were normal findings, they want those findings documented; not just a list of abnormal findings. Part of this preference is the assumption many providers have that if a finding was not mentioned, then the practitioner had either not reviewed the information or had not performed the test (Bosmans et al., 2011). That being said, the most appropriate place for pertinent negative information is probably in the documentation section of the record rather than the report.

In communication with other providers, time is an issue. Being concise in communication and focusing on the conclusions and recommendations of the encounter allows other providers to quickly understand the situation and apply it to their assessment. Forcing another provider to wade through excessively detailed reports creates the risk of the reader missing the most important portions of the communication.

There is often information that is typically normal, or at least congruent, on an audiogram. For example, word recognition performance is typically predictable from the degree and configuration of the hearing loss. However, in instances where there is unusually poor word recognition, retrocochlear pathology may be indicated. It is the audiologist's obligation to make the patient's physician aware of this possibility. If statements about word recognition performance being consistent with the hearing loss are included in a report routinely, the physician reading the report may be trained to filter out this usually unimportant information. By highlighting this information only when its abnormality is potentially diagnostically significant, the reader is provided with a "new" piece of information that is less likely to be missed or ignored.

Another consideration in an encounter involves the need to draw attention to unusual or abnormal results. Physicians receive a large number of reports on their patients in any given day. When sending out information in the form of written reports to providers, it is often helpful to send a follow-up message in the form of an email or telephone call to alert the provider to the fact that an abnormal or unusual report result is coming their way. Most health care providers are grateful for the attention paid to their patient and for the assistance in sorting through the avalanche of information that they must use to make clinical decisions. If a goal of an encounter is conveying to a provider evidence that a patient has signs of retrocochlear dysfunction, and the importance of this evidence is seemingly overlooked by a provider, then the goal has not been met.

❖ Common Language ❖

In addition to the template format for structuring a report, use of consistent language is beneficial in relaying information to other providers. Bosmans and colleagues (2011) found that physician providers preferred a standard lexicon for reporting findings. Findings in audiologic evaluation are often precise, and subtle changes in meaning that occur with variations of language can distort meaning unintentionally. Grieve and colleagues (2010) found that physicians preferred that abbreviations not be included in reports because nonspecialist providers may not understand them, or they may be confused with other abbreviations or acronyms. This is also consistent with the Joint Commission's guidance on the use of abbreviations.

Beginning clinicians are often tempted to convey information in a highly formal manner and may use complicated text. However, complexity of language and grammar in reporting should be kept to a minimum. Information should be described in a way that is straightforward and simple. The words used in a report not only convey content but also convey certain impressions. A study by Sierra and colleagues (1992) found that there was a negative correlation between linguistic complexity and clarity and the impression of certainty of the reporter. This means that the more complicated a description was, the less the reader felt the writer was confident about the findings. Care should be taken to use the most uncomplicated language possible to facilitate communication.

❖ Hearing Evaluation Report ❖

Regardless of the type of report that is formulated, a report of a hearing evaluation generally has common goals and includes specific information. A hearing evaluation report can generally be divided into four areas of assessment: middle ear function, hearing function, retrocochlear function, and communicative function. These would then be followed by the audiologist's plan or recommendations. Consistent with the principle of "getting the order right," the impressions should be summarized at the beginning of the report, followed by the recommendations. Data leading up to these conclusions should be addressed in the documentation section following. To bring the reader's attention to abnormal findings, formatting cues such as bold, colored, or capital lettering can be used where appropriate.

A: Assessment

The four areas of function to include in the audiologic assessment are supported by the audiologic data. These data often overlap in their contribution to functional outcomes. For example, an air-bone gap contributes to both characterizations of middle ear function as well as the type of hearing loss. Word recognition scores support interpretation of hearing sensitivity, retrocochlear function, and communicative function. Acoustic reflex thresholds can be used to support interpretation of middle ear function, hearing function, and retrocochlear function. The audiologist can contribute substantially to the health care team when these data are interpreted for the referring physician and communicated in terms of functional outcomes.

Middle Ear Function

The first question of interest is whether middle ear function is normal or abnormal. If abnormal, characterization of the functional consequences is useful. Note that an assessment of middle ear function is not the same as a recitation of immittance results. An assessment of middle ear function requires interpretation of immittance results and requires collection of data necessary for valid interpretation. Without a complete data set, interpretation is necessarily limited. An example of this is the case of otosclerosis. Early otosclerosis may not demonstrate a significant air-bone gap and may present with a normal tympanogram. Acoustic reflex data would provide a valid interpretation of middle ear function as abnormal. Strength of interpretation regarding middle ear function is increased when immittance findings of tympanometry and acoustic reflex thresholds are supported by type of hearing loss (presence of air-bone gap), tuning fork test outcomes, and otoscopic examination findings. Descriptions for assessment of middle ear function can be found in Table 7–1. It is the descriptions, located in the right-hand column, which would be used in the assessment. The supporting information, in the left-hand column, would be housed in the documentation section of the record.

Table 7–1. Descriptors of Middle Ear Function

Immittance Outcomes	Description of Middle Ear Function
Normal tympanometry and acoustic reflexes	Normal middle ear function
Normal or shallow tympanogram and absent acoustic reflexes (not consistent with degree of hearing sensitivity loss)	Middle ear disorder: Increased stiffness
Type A tympanogram and abnormal acoustic reflex thresholds	Middle ear disorder: Decreased stiffness
Type B tympanogram; absent acoustic reflexes; normal volume	Middle ear disorder: Increased mass
Type B tympanogram with large volume	Middle ear function consistent with a perforation of the tympanic membrane or patent P.E. tube
Abnormal tympanogram and equivalent ear canal volume with a history of ear surgery	Abnormal middle ear function consistent with a history of otologic surgery
Type C tympanogram	Middle ear disorder: Significant negative pressure
Normal tympanograms and acoustic reflexes not performed	Data consistent with normal type A tympanogram. Interpretation of middle ear function limited by lack of acoustic reflex information

Hearing Function

Hearing function can be described using a few vital pieces of information. First, is hearing normal or abnormal? If abnormal, hearing sensitivity should be characterized by defining the type, degree, and configuration of the hearing loss. Judgment should be made as to whether hearing is symmetric between the ears and, if the information is available, whether meaningful change in hearing has occurred over time. Descriptions for assessment of hearing function can be found in Table 7–2.

Table 7–2. Descriptors of Hearing Function

Degree	Normal (−10 to 10 dB)
	Minimal (11 to 25 dB)
	Mild (26 to 40 dB)
	Moderate (41 to 55 dB)
	Moderately severe (56 to 70 dB)
	Severe (71 to 90 dB)
	Profound (>90 dB)
Configuration	High-frequency
	Low-frequency
	Rising
	Flat
Type	Conductive
	Sensorineural
	Mixed
Change Over Time	Sensitivity essentially unchanged since previous evaluation (use specific date if available)
	Sensitivity decreased since previous evaluation (use specific date if available)
	Sensitivity improved since previous evaluation (use specific date if available)
Symmetry	Symmetric
	Asymmetric

Type

The terminology used for describing type of hearing loss should be conductive, sensorineural, or mixed. A hearing loss that is sensorineural at some frequencies and conductive at others should be referred to as a mixed hearing loss. When the patient has a mixed hearing loss, both types of losses can be described to the patient and the patient can typically readily understand that both types are present.

Degree

In describing the degree of hearing loss, the audiologist is providing terminology for patients and family members to understand the severity of hearing loss. This important description will be used by the patient and family members, as well as other health care providers, to draw a host of conclusions about the hearing loss and about the need for intervention for the hearing loss. It is important to be as comprehensible as possible when describing degree of hearing loss to patients. This means being clear as well as concise.

If the hearing loss is essentially flat in configuration, one term that best describes severity should be sufficient. When degree of hearing loss differs over the frequency range, it is of little to no help to patients and to other health care providers to refer to the exact frequencies where crossover between degrees occurs. This information is readily apparent from your audiometric data. However, describing the degree of low-frequency versus high-frequency sounds may be helpful by allowing patients to make sense of their varied and often confusing experiences with hearing loss. For example, such information may help patients understand why they are able to hear male voices better than female voices.

For a hearing loss that is better than 10 dB HL, the term mild loss should be used.

❖ Thresholds of 11 to 25 dB HL are a minimal hearing loss.

❖ A mild hearing loss occurs at 26 to 40 dB HL.

❖ Moderate hearing loss occurs at 41 to 55 dB HL.

❖ Moderately severe hearing loss occurs at 56 to 70 dB HL.

❖ A severe hearing loss is in the range of 71 to 90 dB HL.

❖ A profound hearing loss can be used to describe anything greater than a 90 dB HL loss.

Configuration

The configuration of a hearing loss refers to its general shape on the audiogram. The use of terms to describe shape of the hearing loss helps verbally depict how the hearing varies as a function of frequency. If a reader did not have access to the graphic depiction of the audiogram, the terminology used to describe configuration can be useful in characterizing the hearing loss.

Terminology used to describe the configuration of the hearing loss should be simple and concise. It is helpful to use words that are commonly understood among hearing care professionals and to use this terminology consistently to avoid confusion for patients. The term "flat" refers to a hearing loss that is relatively similar (within about 20 dB or so) among the frequencies tested. The term "sloping" refers to a hearing loss that is better in the low frequencies and then gradually decreases in the high frequencies. A "steeply sloping" hearing loss depicts a hearing loss that is better in the low frequencies and then rapidly decreases in the higher frequencies. A hearing loss that is poorer in the low frequencies and is better in the higher frequencies is known as a "rising" or "reverse slope" hearing loss. If hearing is normal in one frequency range, the terms "high-frequency" or "low-frequency" hearing loss may be used to describe the frequency range where hearing occurs.

Symmetry

Symmetry refers to the degree that bone-conduction thresholds between ears match one another. The symmetry of hearing sensitivity can be important for identifying potential ear-specific pathology, such as VIIIth nerve tumors. Asymmetries related solely to conductive components of a hearing loss are irrelevant for pointing to such potential pathology, and should not be mentioned. The term symmetric may be used when describing hearing loss. Alternatively, when the hearing loss is symmetric this can be considered a normal outcome, which may not require comment. The decision to comment on a hearing loss as asymmetric is important, but it is not simple. Margolis and Saly (2007) reviewed hearing loss data from a large clinical population. Results showed that over half of their patients had asymmetric hearing, if typical criteria for defining asymmetric were used. This finding suggests that relatively small asymmetries in hearing sensitivity may, in fact, be normal. Accordingly, audiologists may wish to take a more conservative view when reporting that a hearing loss is asymmetric. In particular, asymmetric hearing sensitivity should be brought to the attention of the reader when the asymmetry is large or when there are other factors that may point to retrocochlear pathology, such as asymmetric word recognition scores or abnormal acoustic reflex testing results.

Change in Hearing Status

When evaluating hearing, it is important to determine whether a patient has had a previous evaluation and what the results of the evaluation are. Information regarding changes in hearing status over time or stability of hearing over time can be an important component of the diagnostic picture for a patient. In many cases a patient may be seeking periodic hearing evaluations to monitor changes in hearing over time or to screen hearing for employment or other purposes. Particularly in cases of monitoring programs, change from a baseline hearing test must be recognized.

In other cases, hearing evaluation may be recommended to rule out further hearing loss as a contributing factor to difficulty with audiologic intervention. For example, a patient may report greater difficulty than previously with hearing aids, and a hearing evaluation may help explain why this may be occurring.

It may be recommended that patients receive repeated audiologic evaluation to monitor changes in hearing related to disease, medical treatment, or to evaluate effectiveness of medical intervention. For example, a patient with suspected Meniere's disease may require repeated audiologic evaluations to document fluctuations in hearing loss related to the disease process. Patients who undergo treatment with medications known to be ototoxic may undergo repeated evaluations to obtain a baseline evaluation of hearing and to monitor changes over time to determine whether dosage may need to be changed. Patients usually receive audiologic evaluation prior to and following otologic surgery. In this case, improvements in hearing are often the expected outcome, and changes from baseline are important. For patients who receive medical treatment for sudden hearing loss or otitis media, follow-up hearing evaluations are needed to understand the effectiveness of treatment. In all of these cases, comments should be made about the degree of hearing loss during current evaluation compared to previous and baseline evaluations.

Retrocochlear Function

The assessment of the audiologist with regard to retrocochlear function requires a judgment of whether there are audiologic indicators for abnormal retrocochlear function, and if so, a description of the results consistent with dysfunction. This information helps the referring physician determine what additional evaluation, if any, to pursue. Table 7–3 shows descriptions that may be used in assessment of retrocochlear function. In contrast to the assessments

Table 7–3. Descriptors for Retrocochlear Function

Normal: No audiologic indicators of retrocochlear dysfunction

Signs of retrocochlear dysfunction: Acoustic reflex thresholds are abnormally elevated

Signs of retrocochlear dysfunction: Reflex decay testing shows significant auditory adaptation

Signs of retrocochlear dysfunction: Word-recognition score is significantly poorer than expected from the hearing loss

Signs of retrocochlear dysfunction: Word-recognition testing shows significant rollover

Signs of retrocochlear dysfunction: Asymmetric signs (hearing sensitivity, word recognition) and symptoms (tinnitus, etc.)

of middle ear function and hearing-sensitivity function, the terminology used in these exams includes some data in a more raw form. This is because, in most cases, when a physician is confronted with evidence for retrocochlear dysfunction, he or she often relies on a summarization of these data to determine the strength of the evidence for retrocochlear dysfunction in determining next steps to take. For example, relatively minor signs may sway a physician one way, such as observation and reevaluation, whereas more pronounced signs may sway the physician toward other plans, such as auditory brainstem evaluation or magnetic resonance imaging.

Communicative Function

The fourth major component of the assessment is communicative function. Communicative function refers to how well patients are able to communicate given their hearing loss and ability to understand speech. This concept also takes into account the patients' self-reported function, which is influenced by his or her abilities to compensate for hearing deficits and their unique personal communication demands. An assessment of communicative function is needed in cases where there is concern for whether the patient may be in need of audiologic intervention. A referring physician will want to understand if the patient is a candidate for audiologic treatment. Descriptions that may be used in describing communicative function can be found in Table 7–4 for adults and Table 7–5 for children.

P: Plan

Recommendations are based on the patient's history, behavioral and objective audiometric findings, communication impact, patient and family reports of need, and preferences regarding potential audiologic intervention. Whether patients, families, and other medical providers agree with the judgment of the audiologist regarding hearing health care recommendations, it is the responsibility of the audiologist to provide recommendations based on the aforementioned factors.

Table 7–4. Descriptors of Communicative Function for Adults

Adults

Normal

Mild dysfunction: Hearing sensitivity loss sufficient to impair speech perception, particularly in noisy situations. However, patient reports little to no difficulty.

Mild dysfunction: Minimal hearing sensitivity loss. However, patient reports difficulty, particularly in noisy situations.

Mild dysfunction: Normal/minimal hearing sensitivity loss. Understanding of speech poorer than expected for degree of hearing loss. Patient reports difficulty.

Mild dysfunction with treatment: Hearing sensitivity loss sufficient to impair speech perception when left untreated. However, patient's consistent use of hearing amplification and/or assistive technology provides sufficient benefit for acceptable communication function.

Moderate dysfunction: Hearing sensitivity loss sufficient to impair speech perception in both quiet and noisy situations. However, patient reports little difficulty.

Moderate dysfunction: Hearing sensitivity loss sufficient to impair speech perception in both quiet and noisy situations. Patient reports little/moderate difficulty.

Moderate dysfunction: Hearing sensitivity loss sufficient to mildly impair speech perception. However, understanding of speech poorer than expected for degree of hearing loss. Patient reports difficulty.

Moderate dysfunction with treatment: Hearing sensitivity loss sufficient to moderately impair speech perception when left untreated. Patient's use of hearing amplification and/or assistive technology has been inconsistent/has not provided sufficient benefit for acceptable communication function.

Severe dysfunction: Hearing sensitivity loss sufficient to significantly impair speech perception. Patient reports little/moderate/significant difficulty.

Severe dysfunction with treatment: Hearing sensitivity loss sufficient to severely impair speech perception when left untreated. Patient's use of hearing amplification and/or assistive technology has been insufficient for acceptable communication function.

Table 7–5. Descriptors of Communicative Function for Children

Pediatrics

Normal: Hearing sufficient for normal speech and language development.

Mild dysfunction: Hearing sensitivity loss sufficient to impair speech perception, particularly in noisy situations. Patient at risk for impaired speech and language development; however, no known current speech and language delay.

Mild dysfunction with treatment. Hearing sensitivity loss sufficient to impair speech perception, particularly in noisy situations if left untreated. However, patient's consistent use of hearing amplification and/or assistive technology provides sufficient benefit for acceptable communication function.

Moderate dysfunction: Hearing sensitivity loss sufficient to impair speech perception in both quiet and noisy situations. Patient at heightened risk for impaired speech and language development; however, no known current speech and language delay.

Moderate dysfunction: Hearing sensitivity loss sufficient to impair speech perception. Known speech and language delay.

Severe dysfunction: Hearing sensitivity loss sufficient to severely impair speech perception when left untreated. Patient at high risk for impaired speech and language development. Known speech and language delay.

Severe dysfunction with treatment: Hearing sensitivity loss sufficient to severely impair speech perception when left untreated. Patient at high risk for impaired speech and language development. Known speech and language delay. Patient's use of hearing amplification and/or assistive technology has been insufficient for acceptable communication function.

What To Do With Speech Audiometry Results?

Description of speech audiometric results can be used to supplement description of pure-tone audiometric findings. In the vast majority of cases, speech audiometric results are consistent with the pure-tone audiogram. That is, speech recognition thresholds are within about 7 decibels of the 3-tone pure-tone average at 500, 1,000, and 2,000 Hz, and the word recognition scores fall within a range of values that are predicted from the degree and configuration of hearing loss. As such, the most commonly used speech audiometric results do not provide additional information to the reader about hearing status. Although speech audiometric scores must be documented in the hearing evaluation results, it is our recommendation that when speech recognition thresholds and word recognition thresholds are consistent with the pure-tone audiogram, these results should not be included in the reporting section of the record. Consistent repetition of the phrase "speech audiometric results consistent with audiogram" is likely to train even the most interested and discerning reader to gloss over these results, potentially causing the reader to miss important information when the results are not predictable. Rather than focusing on an interpretation of these results in and of themselves, they should be placed into the context of their role in function, such as retrocochlear or communicative function.

One case in which speech audiometric results may differ from expectations is when speech recognition thresholds do not agree with the pure-tone thresholds. When such results cannot be explained by hearing loss configuration or some other factor, suspicion should be raised about functional hearing loss. In this case, it is important to note in the hearing test results that there is inconsistency between pure-tone and speech threshold measures.

When word recognition scores deviate significantly from what is predicted from the hearing loss, speech audiometric results become an important component of the diagnosis picture. In some cases, rollover of the performance/intensity function may even be observed. In either case, the discrepancy between the expected and obtained results should be highlighted in describing the hearing evaluation outcomes.

In some cases of symmetric hearing, word recognition scores can be significantly different between ears, raising suspicion of retrocochlear dysfunction. In this case, the asymmetric word recognition scores should be highlighted in the results.

For some individuals, binaural word recognition results may demonstrate poorer performance in a binaural compared to monaural condition. This outcome suggests the presence of binaural interference, which has important implications for audiologic intervention. Such anomalies should be highlighted in the results.

When describing discrepancies between pure-tone and speech-recognition scores, the phrase "speech recognition poorer than expected for degree of hearing loss" can be used. In describing word recognition scores that raise concern for retrocochlear dysfunction, such as unexpectedly poor scores, rollover of the performance/intensity function, or asymmetric scores, the phrase "word recognition scores consistent with retrocochlear dysfunction" may be used. When binaural scores are poorer than single ear scores, the phrase "word recognition scores consistent with binaural interference" may be used.

In many cases, patients are referred to an audiologist for a consultation regarding hearing function. It is always most appropriate to refer the patient back to the referring physician for follow-up care regarding hearing and ear function. In other cases, patients may present to an audiologist on their own for any number of reasons. Should the audiologic examination demonstrate any indication of potential external ear disorder, middle ear disorder, or retrocochlear dysfunction, referral to a primary care physician or otolaryngologist should be made. In cases of stable sensorineural hearing loss where audiologic intervention including hearing aids, cochlear implant, or other implant evaluation is indicated, referral should be made to a physician for medical clearance for hearing aids or consultation for surgical candidacy for implantation.

Children who are referred for hearing evaluation often have an additional set of concerns related to hearing loss that may result in additional recommendations for professional evaluation. Some children are referred for hearing evaluation due to concerns about speech and/or language development. When audiologic evaluation results demonstrate that hearing is sufficient for speech and language development, recommendation may be made for evaluation by a speech-language pathologist. When a child is identified with a hearing loss, there is often a need to refer for additional educational intervention services. Referral may be appropriate to early intervention programs and/or to the appropriate school personnel for habilitative services in the school system.

During the course of evaluation of hearing, the need for additional diagnostic measures within the scope of audiology may be identified. In these cases, it is appropriate to recommend to the referring physician that further diagnostic testing may be useful based on case history and hearing test outcomes. Recommendations for electrophysiology measures, balance function testing, and auditory processing evaluation may be made. In addition, further evaluation of hearing may be indicated depending on the needs identified by the audiologist.

All patients should be routinely cautioned against exposure to excessively loud noise. In some cases, patients may admit to behaviors that put hearing at risk or may show evidence of noise induced hearing loss in the audiologic evaluation results. For these patients in particular, formal recommendation for use of hearing protection in noise should be made.

Recommendations for audiologic intervention should also be made at the time of hearing evaluation. If hearing loss is of a severity suggesting that hearing instruments may be beneficial, recommendation should be made for a hearing aid evaluation. If other amplification or assistive listening devices are clearly indicated at the time of hearing evaluation, these should be mentioned as well. When providing recommendation for hearing instrument evaluation, it is appropriate to identify cases when the patient is clearly a candidate for binaural or single ear amplification. For patients who have contraindications for binaural amplification, such as binaural interference, extremely poor word recognition in one ear, medical contraindications for aiding a particular ear, or any other factors that would contraindicate binaural amplification, recommendations for unilateral amplification should be indicated. If a patient is a candidate for special types of hearing instrumentation, such as a CROS or BICROS system, this information should be included in the recommendation as well.

For patients whose hearing and word recognition is too poor to benefit effectively from hearing instruments, a cochlear implant evaluation should be considered and recommendations made when appropriate. Patients who are potential candidates for osseointegrated bone conduction devices should be identified and recommendations made for evaluation when appropriate. For patients who have identified problems with tinnitus, evaluation for potential treatment of tinnitus may be an appropriate recommendation as well. Descriptions of potential recommendations can be found in Table 7–6.

Table 7–6. Descriptors of Potential Audiologic Recommendations

No additional audiologic recommendations.

Medical consultation for evaluation of middle ear disorder.

Recommendations deferred pending otologic consultation.

Audiometric exam following completion of medical management.

Continued monitoring of hearing sensitivity (annually, 6 months, etc.).

If additional audiologic diagnostic information is needed, consider auditory brainstem response testing.

If additional audiologic diagnostic information is needed, consider balance function testing.

Evoked response audiometry to further assess hearing sensitivity.

Hearing aid selection following medical clearance.

Cochlear implant evaluation.

Evaluation for osseointegrated device.

❖ Electrophysiology Reports ❖

The goals for reporting of electrophysiology results depend upon the purpose for which the test was recommended. For diagnostic auditory brainstem response testing, the report should clearly state whether results were normal or abnormal. Abnormal results can be further explained to demonstrate evidence of VIIIth nerve dysfunction. Details documenting the testing protocol and results should be included following the interpretation or included as an addendum to the report. Some examples of descriptors for diagnostic auditory brainstem response evaluation can be found in Table 7–7.

For threshold prediction auditory brainstem response or auditory steady-state response testing, the report should provide a clear statement of the hearing sensitivity predicted by the measures. If hearing loss exists, statement about the degree and type of hearing loss should be made. Recommendations should be provided for follow-up when this is necessary. If electrophysiologic measures are used for screening of hearing, a clear statement of pass or refer should be provided. For threshold prediction measures in patients

Table 7–7. Descriptors for Diagnostic Auditory Brainstem Response Evaluation

---

ABR shows well-formed responses to click stimuli at normal absolute latencies and interwave intervals. There is no electrophysiologic evidence of VIIIn or auditory brainstem pathway disorder.

ABR shows abnormal responses to click stimuli. Both the absolute latency of wave V and the I to V interwave interval are significantly prolonged. These results are consistent with VIIIn or auditory brainstem pathway disorder.

ABR shows responses to click stimuli at absolute latencies consistent with the peripheral hearing loss. There is no electrophysiologic evidence of VIIIn or auditory brainstem pathway disorder.

---

on whom behavioral measures have been obtained, statements should be made regarding agreement between the objective and behavioral measures. Terminology for threshold prediction should be similar to those used to describe behavioral thresolds. Examples can be found in Table 7–2.

❖ Auditory Processing Reports ❖

The goal for reports of auditory processing evaluation is to convey to the reader the functional deficit for the patient in terms of suprathreshold hearing and to provide understandable recommendations for treatment. The report should provide a diagnosis of whether auditory processing disorder exists, what specific areas of deficit were found, and what recommendations have been provided to the patient. Data documenting the tests utilized and the outcomes of tests should be included following this information, or as an addendum to the report. Although it is helpful to the reader to provide a succinct description of the testing protocols utilized in the documentation section, it is unnecessary to describe the tests in detail. Examples of descriptions of auditory processing evaluation assessments and recommendations can be found in Table 7–8.

Table 7–8. Examples of Descriptions for Auditory Processing Evaluation and Recommendations

Normal suprathreshold auditory function.
Auditory processing disorder characterized by reduced speech perception bilaterally at high intensity levels, with poorer performance on the right ear.
The patient would likely benefit from mild gain hearing aid amplification, with better prognosis if fitted on the left ear.
The patient would likely benefit from remote microphone technology in the classroom situation.

❖ Functional Hearing Loss ❖

In the case of suspected functional hearing loss, the final version of the hearing test results should reflect only the results deemed to be accurate. More about documentation of the specific results was described in the previous chapter. For the assessment component of such a case, the phrases, "consistent results unable to be obtained" or "behavioral measures inconsistent with objective measures" as appropriate will clearly communicate that the outcomes are not as expected and that no additional information can be obtained. However, any objective data that can be interpreted should be. For example, in the presence of robust otoacoustic emissions and normal acoustic reflex thresholds, the phrase, "objective measures are consistent with no greater than mild sensorineural hearing loss" can be used to provide an assessment of hearing sensitivity. The plan component of the record may include reevaluation using behavioral measures, evaluation using electrophysiologic measures for threshold prediction, or other appropriate follow-up.

CHAPTER 8

Sample Reporting and Documentation

In this final chapter, we present examples of reporting and documentation across a variety of clinical applications. As we alluded to throughout this text, the exact format and style of reporting varies widely across clinics and is often dictated to a substantial extent by requirements or preferences of a given setting and institution. In fact, it is doubtful that most of us could even reach consensus on the wording to be used within a given report, and it is probably unnecessary to do so. However, there are general rules that should be considered in refining your strategy for reporting. These have been detailed in previous chapters but are worth remembering as you review these examples. When documenting and reporting you should:

❖ get to the point quickly;

❖ don't make the reader work for the answer;

❖ write less, not more;

❖ use consistent language whenever possible;

❖ state outcomes, recommendations, and dispositions clearly;

❖ get the order right;

❖ report first, then document;

❖ distinguish important information; and

❖ include only relevant information.

With those general rules as a guide, following are examples of reports commonly used in a clinical audiology setting. Some of the reports are designed to convey clinical outcomes to patients and providers. Others are designed simply to document an outcome or an encounter. Most, however, both document clinical outcomes and convey a summary of that documentation to the interested reader.

❖ Hearing Evaluation Report and Documentation ❖

The following examples combine reporting and documentation from the electronic medical records system used at the Henry Ford Hospital in Detroit, Michigan. A tablet-based software app, known as eAudio™, is used to input data collected from the entire encounter, including history, otoscopic examination, immittance measures, and pure-tone and speech audiometry. Results are interpreted and summarized using drop-down menus, and the resultant report is sent wirelessly to the patient's file within Henry Ford Hospital's electronic medical record (EMR) system.

The reports are designed to provide the chief complaint, a summary of the audiometric assessment, and the recommendations before the presentation of any data. Audiometric data are then presented in the order of probable importance to the reader, followed eventually by the fine detail of documentation. Figure 8–1 is an example of the outcome of an adult diagnostic assessment. These results were obtained on a 60-year-old woman with a chief complaint of bilateral hearing loss. For privacy purposes, her results were uploaded into a "dummy" patient file in the EMR system under the name "Wilma Flintstone." She was found to have bilateral, symmetric sensorineural hearing loss and was interested in pursuing hearing aid use. She was referred to an otolaryngologist for medical clearance and referred for a hearing aid selection.

Figure 8–2 is an example of the outcome of a pediatric diagnostic assessment. These results were obtained from a 3-year-old girl whose parents were concerned with hearing loss. For privacy purposes, her results were uploaded into a "dummy" patient file in the EMR system under the name "Pebbles Flintstone." She was found to have bilateral middle ear disorder and conductive hearing loss. She was referred for otologic consultation.

Henry Ford Health System: Division of Audiology
MRN: 52424608
Patient Name: Wilma Flintstone **SEX:** female
DOB: 12/6/1952 (60yrs old)
Associated ENT Not specified
Referring Physician Not specified
Exam performed by: VirginiaRamachandran, Au.D., Ph.D.
Exam Date: 1/3/2013

CHIEF COMPLAINT

- Right ear has hearing loss
- Left ear has hearing loss

SUMMARY

RIGHT
- Mild sloping to Moderate-severe high-frequency sensorineural hearing loss
- Acoustic immittance measures are consistent with normal middle ear function

LEFT
- Mild sloping to Moderate-severe high-frequency sensorineural hearing loss
- Acoustic immittance measures are consistent with normal middle ear function

RECOMMENDATIONS

- To ENT appointment as planned
- Schedule Hearing Aid Selection

AUDIOGRAM

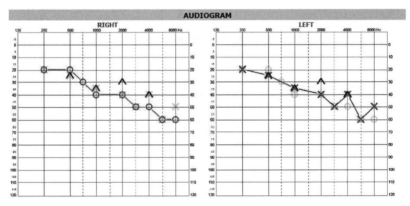

PTA:33 SRT:35   PTA:33 SRT:35

Word Recognition

Air Conduction   100 % at 80 dBHL   Air Conduction   96 % at 80 dBHL

	AIR CONDUCTION (A/C)		BONE CONDUCTION (B/C)			No Response	Sound Field	S
	Unmasked	Masked	Unmasked	Masked	Unspecified		Aided	A
R	O	Δ	<	[	∧	◇	Could Not Test	CNT
L	X	□	>	]		◇	Did Not Test	DNT

Figure 8–1. *continues*

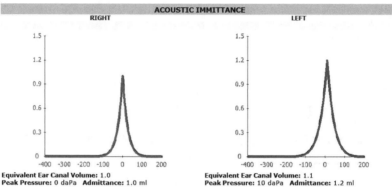

ACOUSTIC IMMITTANCE

RIGHT

Equivalent Ear Canal Volume: 1.0
Peak Pressure: 0 daPa   Admittance: 1.0 ml

Acoustic Reflex Thresholds

	BBN	500Hz	1000Hz	2000Hz
Ipsilateral (probe right - sound right)			85 dBHL	90 dBHL
Contralateral (probe left - sound right)	85 dBHL	95 dBHL	90 dBHL	85 dBHL

Contra Stimulus / Reflex Decay:500Hz: (-)   1000Hz: (-)

LEFT

Equivalent Ear Canal Volume: 1.1
Peak Pressure: 10 daPa   Admittance: 1.2 ml

Acoustic Reflex Thresholds

	BBN	500Hz	1000Hz	2000Hz
Ipsilateral (probe left - sound left)			80 dBHL	85 dBHL
Contralateral (probe right - sound left)	85 dBHL	90 dBHL	95 dBHL	90 dBHL

Contra Stimulus / Reflex Decay:500Hz: (-)   1000Hz: (-)

SPEECH THRESHOLDS

RIGHT

Air Conduction: 35
SRT Spondees, MLV, Insert Phones

LEFT

Air Conduction: 35
SRT Spondees, MLV, Insert Phones

WORD RECOGNITION DETAILS

	RIGHT	LEFT
Air Conduction Test 1	Masked 80 dBHL 100 % NU-6 Rank Order list 1 Recorded / Inserts	Masked 80 dBHL 96 % NU-6 Rank Order list 2 Recorded / Inserts

CASE HISTORY DETAILS

Right ear has hearing loss.
Left ear has hearing loss.
Onset: Gradually over 10 years

Right ear has tinnitus.
Sounds like: Ringing
Left ear has tinnitus.
Sounds like: Ringing
Onset: Unknown

Right ear has: Pressure

Family history of hearing loss: No
Do you wear hearing aids? No

Testing completed after excessive cerumen removed: Right and Left

Patient reliability is Good
Location: Main Campus
History given by: Patient
The patient does NOT report dizziness.
This is NOT a post-medical management or surgery visit.
The patient has reportedly NOT been exposed to loud noise.

Figure 8–1. *continued*

Henry Ford Health System: Division of Audiology
MRN: 56662436
Patient Name: Pebbles Flintstone **SEX:** female
DOB: 1/22/2009 (3yrs old)
Associated ENT Not specified
Referring Physician Not specified
Exam performed by: VirginiaRamachandran, Au.D., Ph.D.
Exam Date: 1/3/2013

CHIEF COMPLAINT

- Right ear has hearing loss
- Left ear has hearing loss

SUMMARY

RIGHT

- Mild conductive hearing loss
- Acoustic immittance measures indicate a middle ear disorder; Flat, Type B tympanogram consistent with increased mass of the middle ear mechanism

LEFT

- Mild conductive hearing loss
- Acoustic immittance measures indicate a middle ear disorder; Flat, Type B tympanogram consistent with increased mass of the middle ear mechanism

RECOMMENDATIONS

- To ENT appointment as planned
- Retest post medical management, if any

AUDIOGRAM

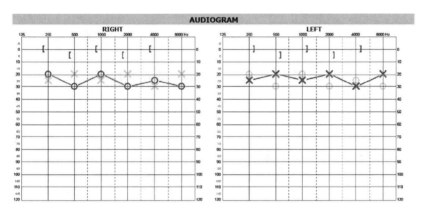

PTA:27 SRT:30   PTA:22 SRT:25

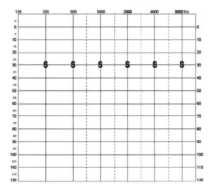

Figure 8–2. *continues*

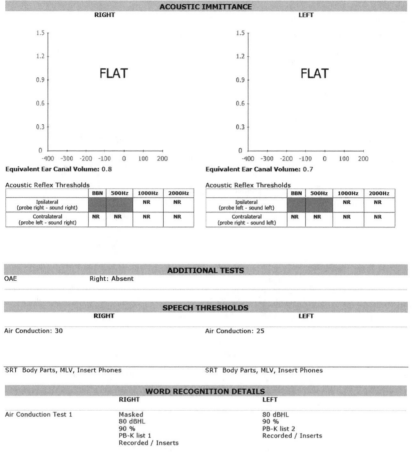

ACOUSTIC IMMITTANCE

RIGHT

FLAT

Equivalent Ear Canal Volume: 0.8

Acoustic Reflex Thresholds

	BBN	500Hz	1000Hz	2000Hz
Ipsilateral (probe right - sound right)			NR	NR
Contralateral (probe left - sound right)	NR	NR	NR	NR

LEFT

FLAT

Equivalent Ear Canal Volume: 0.7

Acoustic Reflex Thresholds

	BBN	500Hz	1000Hz	2000Hz
Ipsilateral (probe left - sound left)			NR	NR
Contralateral (probe right - sound left)	NR	NR	NR	NR

ADDITIONAL TESTS

OAE   Right: Absent

SPEECH THRESHOLDS

RIGHT   LEFT

Air Conduction: 30   Air Conduction: 25

SRT Body Parts, MLV, Insert Phones   SRT Body Parts, MLV, Insert Phones

WORD RECOGNITION DETAILS

	RIGHT	LEFT
Air Conduction Test 1	Masked 80 dBHL 90 % PB-K list 1 Recorded / Inserts	80 dBHL 90 % PB-K list 2 Recorded / Inserts

CASE HISTORY DETAILS

Right ear has hearing loss.
Left ear has hearing loss.
Onset: Off and on with reported ear infections.

Right ear has: Pain

Family history of hearing loss: No
Do you wear hearing aids? No

Normal Pregnancy: Yes
Prematurity: No
Hearing screening at birth: Yes Pass
Does the child have any risk factors for hearing loss: No
Family history of childhood or progressive hearing loss: No
Parental concerns with hearing: Yes
Parental concerns with speech/language: No
School performance concerns: No

Patient reliability is Good
Location: Main Campus
History given by: Mother
The patient does NOT report tinnitus.
The patient does NOT report dizziness.
The patient has reportedly NOT been exposed to loud noise.

Figure 8–2. *continued*

❖ Hearing Instrument Report and Documentation ❖

Following are four examples of the types of reporting and documentation used for hearing aid patients at the Henry Ford Hospital in Detroit, Michigan. A report is made at the time of hearing aid selection, and another is made at the time of hearing aid delivery and orientation. A progress note is included in the electronic medical record at every follow-up encounter, whether in person or by phone. Finally, a sequential list of encounters is maintained as "encounter notes" to track the patient's progress with hearing aid amplification.

Hearing aid reports are designed differently than diagnostic reports because of the nature of the information and the nature of who will be reading them. Records kept for most hearing aid encounters serve the purpose of documenting more than reporting. They are most likely to be read by the audiologist providing ongoing care or by technical and support staff who might be assisting.

Figure 8–3 is an example of the outcome of a hearing aid selection. Here, the specifics of the devices are documented, along with the verification of medical clearance. Also included is the rationale for the selection, which can be a reminder to the audiologist of why certain decisions were made at the time of selection.

Figure 8–4 is an example of a record that can be used to document and report the outcome of hearing aid delivery and orientation. Here, the specifics of the devices are documented, along with the verification of the actual hearing aid fit. Also included is a summary of the orientation of the patient to the devices and documentation of a follow-up appointment.

Figure 8–5 is an example of a short summary note used to document a hearing aid follow-up appointment or any subsequent patient encounter. This serves as a summary of why the patient sought care, what was accomplished during the encounter, and a clear statement of the disposition.

Figure 8–6 is an example of patient encounter notes used with hearing aid patients. These notes are a brief summary of encounters, listed sequentially, that provide the audiologist or technical staff with a perspective of the patient's overall history of his or her experience with hearing aid devices.

HEARING AID SELECTION

Right:
Manufacturer: Company
Model: Device
Style: Full shell
Color: Medium brown

Left:
Manufacturer: Company
Model: Device
Style: Full shell
Color: Medium brown

SETTINGS AND/OR FEATURES:
Manual programs: None
Adaptation level: 3

MEDICAL CLEARANCE FROM:
Physician: Dr. P. Care
Date: August 14, 2013

RATIONALE:
Binaural amplification is recommended for the patient because the patient has hearing loss in both ears that can be benefited by amplification.

The full shell style of amplification is recommended because of the degree of hearing loss and because of ease of insertion and removal.

Level 1 technology level is recommended because the patient reports being in quiet most of the time.

RETURN APPOINTMENT DATE: September 4, 2013

Figure 8–3.

HEARING AID DELIVERY AND ORIENTATION

The patient was seen today for the delivery and orientation of the new hearing aids coupled to the right and left ears.

Right:
Manufacturer:
Model:
Style:
Color:
Serial Number:

Left:
Manufacturer:
Model:
Style:
Color:
Serial Number:

Electroacoustical analysis of the hearing aids indicates the instruments are functioning within manufacturer's specifications.

Probe tube measurements were consistent with those results expected from the hearing aids.

The patient was counseled relative to the proper use, care, and maintenance of the hearing aids. The patient's initial subjective opinion of the hearing aid was positive.

The patient read the "Hearing Aid Receipt and Warranty Information" form and agreed to its contents by signing the form.

COMMENTS:

• Patient is to return for a hearing aid recheck on.

Figure 8–4.

Hearing Instrument Progress Note

Mr. Green was seen today at the hearing aid walk-in clinic. The patient had a complaint of the right hearing aid not working. Listening check revealed the aid to be weak. The microphone and receiver tube of the hearing aid were cleaned. The listening check was then good and the patient reported that the sound was much better. Performance was confirmed with electroacoustic analysis measures. The patient was reinstructed in cleaning and maintenance of the hearing aid. He will return as needed.

Figure 8–5.

Patient Encounter Notes

Patient Name: **John Doe**

Phone: **313-555-5555**

Date	Notes
1/2/2009	Hearing aid selection appointment. Patient chose hearing aids.
1/14/2009	Hearing aids delivered from manufacturer and checked-in.
	was performed and aids are meeting specifications.
1/20/2009	Hearing aid delivery and orientation appointment. Hearing
	paid in full for the cost of the aids and professional service
1/31/2009	Conformity check appointment. Patient doing well with the
	regarding communication strategies in noisy situations.
	maintenance of the aids. The patient will return in 6 months
7/20/2009	Hearing aid check appointment. The patient was concerned
	of hearing aids. Visual inspection revealed cerumen occlusion
	aids were cleaned and listening check was good.
	demonstrated appropriate hearing aid function. The patient is
	performance of aids. The patient will return as needed.
9/3/2009	Walk-in. The patient dropped off left hearing aid with
	"dead". Listening check confirmed no hearing aid output.
	Performed in-office were unsuccessful. Hearing aid was sent
9/20/2009	Hearing aid returned from repair. Receiver was replaced.
	demonstrated aid was meeting specifications. Hearing aid re-
	patient settings. Patient contacted to pick up hearing aid.

Figure 8–6.

❖ Auditory Electrophysiologic Testing Reports ❖

The following four examples are a combination of reporting and documentation used at the Henry Ford Hospital in Detroit, Michigan, to summarize outcomes from auditory electrophysiologic testing. The first two are reports of diagnostic auditory brainstem response (ABR) testing in adult patients (Figures 8–7 and 8–8). The third is an example of auditory brainstem response testing for follow-up of infants who did not pass their initial hearing screening at birth (Figure 8–9). The fourth is an example of the report used for electrophysiologic threshold prediction of hearing in a pediatric patient (Figure 8–10).

Report of Auditory Brainstem Response Test
Division of Audiology

Auditory brainstem response testing was carried out on May 29, 2013.

Interpretation of Findings:

ABR shows well-formed responses to click stimuli at normal absolute latencies and interwave intervals. There is no electrophysiological evidence of VIIIn or auditory brainstem pathway disorder.

Results:

Click stimuli of alternating polarity, presented at a rate of 21.1/s at 85 dB nHL were used to obtain the following results:

Absolute Latency (msec)	I	III	V
Right	1.92	4.00	6.09
Left	1.96	3.92	6.13

Interwave Intervals (msec)	I-III	III-V	I-V
Right	2.08	2.09	4.17
Left	1.96	2.21	4.17

Interwave Ear Difference (msec)	I-III	III-V	I-V
Right - Left	0.12	-0.12	0.00

Fast Rate Latency (msec)	V fast	V slow	Diff
Right	7.00	6.09	0.91
Left	7.17	6.13	1.04

Amplitude (uV)	I	V	V/I
Right	0.23	0.33	1.43
Left	0.22	0.29	1.32

Audiology Extern:
Senior Staff Audiologist:

Figure 8–7.

```
Report of Auditory Brainstem Response Test
Division of Audiology

Auditory brainstem response testing was carried out on May 29, 2013.

Interpretation of Findings:

ABR shows abnormal responses to click stimuli on the right ear. Both
the absolute latency of wave V and the I to V interwave interval are
significantly prolonged on the right in comparison to the left. These
results are consistent with VIIIn or auditory brainstem pathway
disorder.

Results:

Click stimuli of rarefaction polarity, presented at a rate of 21.1/s at
85 dB nHL were used to obtain the following results:
```

Absolute Latency (msec)	I	III	V
Right	1.50	4.00	5.92
Left	1.54	3.68	5.54

Interwave Intervals (msec)	I-III	III-V	I-V
Right	2.50	1.92	4.42
Left	2.14	1.86	4.00

Interwave Ear Difference (msec)	I-III	III-V	I-V
Right - Left	0.36	0.06	0.42

Fast Rate Latency (msec)	V fast	V slow	Diff
Right	6.25	5.92	0.33
Left	5.92	5.54	0.38

Amplitude (uV)	I	V	V/I
Right	0.31	0.21	0.68
Left	0.27	0.14	0.52

```
Audiology Extern:
Senior Staff Audiologist:
```

Figure 8–8.

The diagnostic ABR reports are designed to provide the outcome and summary before the presentation of any data or of how those data were obtained. Most diagnostic ABR testing is referred by a physician trying to decide whether additional testing is needed to rule out nervous-system disorder. Most referral sources are interested in knowing whether the results are normal or abnormal, not the nuances of how the conclusions were reached. The record, then, is designed to summarize first, with details to follow.

The infant hearing rescreening report is designed much like the diagnostic ABR report, and for the same reason. It is designed to provide a brief history of why the patient is being evaluated,

```
┌─────────────────────────────────────────────────────────────────┐
│                                                                   │
│  Infant Hearing Screening                                         │
│                                                                   │
│  A follow-up hearing screening was completed on June 1, 2013. This │
│  patient had passed a hearing screening on the right ear and failed on │
│  the left ear at birth.                                           │
│                                                                   │
│  Interpretation of Findings:                                      │
│                                                                   │
│  This patient passed the hearing re-screening measures in both ears. │
│                                                                   │
│  Recommendations:                                                 │
│                                                                   │
│  No further audiologic recommendations are indicated at this time. │
│                                                                   │
│  Results:                                                         │
│                                                                   │
│    Right Ear:                                                     │
│                                                                   │
│    Repeatable auditory brainstem responses (ABRs) were recorded at 55 │
│    dB (Wave V latency = 8.12 msec) and 25 dB (9.05 msec).         │
│                                                                   │
│    Left Ear:                                                      │
│                                                                   │
│    Repeatable ABRs were recorded at 55 dB (Wave V latency = 8.12 msec) │
│    and 25 dB (9.05 msec).                                         │
│                                                                   │
│  Audiology Extern:                                                │
│  Senior Staff Audiologist:                                        │
│                                                                   │
└─────────────────────────────────────────────────────────────────┘
```

Figure 8–9.

followed by the outcome and summary, and, finally, by the presentation of data or how those data were obtained. Most infant hearing rescreening reports will be read by pediatricians or members of their staffs. They are interested in knowing whether the results are normal or abnormal, not the nuances of how the conclusions were reached. The record, then, is designed to summarize first, with details to follow. Figure 8–9 is an example of the outcome of infant hearing rescreening in a patient with a normal outcome. In this case, a comment is made at the end that no further audiologic testing is indicated to inform the pediatrician that no additional referrals to audiology are necessary for routine care.

The report used to summarize electrophysiologic threshold prediction is designed like a standard audiometric report, with a summary and recommendations at the beginning and details of how those conclusions were reached to follow. Figure 8–10 is an example of a report that summarizes the use of auditory evoked potentials, otoacoustic emissions, and immittance measures in a patient with conductive hearing loss on one ear and sensorineural hearing loss on the other.

Pediatric Audiologic Consultation

An audiologic consultation was completed on June 1, 2013.

Interpretation of Findings:

The overall pattern of results is consistent with a mild conductive hearing loss and middle ear disorder on the left ear and severe sensorineural hearing loss on the right ear.

Recommendations:

We recommend medical consultation for evaluation of middle ear disorder and sensorineural hearing loss. We recommend audiologic re-evaluation following completion of medical management.

Results:

   Right Ear:

   Auditory brainstem response (ABR) audiometry shows responses to click stimuli down to 85 dB nHL by air conduction. No responses were observed at equipment limits by masked bone conduction. This is consistent with a severe hearing loss in the 1000 to 4000 Hz frequency range.

   Distortion-product otoacoustic emissions (DPOAEs) are absent.

   Tympanometry, obtained with a 1000 Hz probe tone, yielded a normal, Type A tympanogram.

   Left Ear:

   ABR) audiometry shows responses to click stimuli down to 40 dB nHL by air conduction and down to 5 dB nHL by bone conduction. This is consistent with a mild hearing loss in the 1000 to 4000 Hz frequency range.

   Distortion-product otoacoustic emissions (DPOAEs) are absent.

   Acoustic immittance measures indicate middle ear disorder. Tympanometry, obtained with a 1000 Hz probe tone, yielded a flat, Type B tympanogram, consistent with a significant increase in the mass of the middle ear mechanism.

Audiology Extern:
Senior Staff Audiologist:

Figure 8–10.

❖ Auditory Processing Evaluation Report ❖

Following is an example of a combination of reporting and documentation used at the Henry Ford Hospital in Detroit, Michigan, to summarize outcomes from assessment of auditory processing disorder (APD).

The APD report resembles the other diagnostic reports in that the outcome and summary are presented before any data are obtained. As in other diagnostic referrals, most referral sources are interested in knowing whether the results are normal or abnormal, not the nuances of how the conclusions were reached. The record is designed to summarize first, with details to follow. Figure 8–11 is an example of the outcome of diagnostic APD testing in a patient with an abnormal outcome.

The examples are intended to provide some sense of how the principles of reporting and documenting can be put into action. Of course, no set of examples could cover every contingency. By critically thinking about your reporting and documenting methods, you will achieve your intended outcomes of successful communication.

Suprathreshold Hearing Assessment

Suprathreshold hearing assessment was carried out on June 1, 2013 to evaluate auditory processing capabilities.

Interpretation of Findings:

The overall pattern of results is consistent with auditory processing disorder, characterized by reduced speech perception at high intensity levels bilaterally.

Recommendations:

Children with auditory processing disorders of this nature will have difficulty with spatial hearing, particularly in the presence of background noise. We recommend environmental alteration in the classroom and at home to minimize background noise, maximize signal-to-noise ratio, control reverberation, and reinforce audition with visual cues. Remote-microphone technology is indicated if environmental alteration is inadequate to address the child's needs.

Results:

Performance on a test of sentence recognition in the presence of ipsilateral speech competition (Synthetic Sentence Identification test) showed reduced performance bilaterally at 0 dB signal-to-noise ratio:

Left Ear		Right Ear	
100%	60 dB HL	100%	60 dB HL
90%	70 dB HL	90%	70 dB HL
70%	80 dB HL	60%	80 dB HL

Performance on a test of dichotic listening (Dichotic Sentence Identification test), carried out at 70 dB HL with directed attention to one ear, showed a slight right-ear deficit:

Right Ear:	70%
Left Ear:	90%

Performance on a test of temporal resolution (Gaps-in-Noise test), carried out at 50 dB SL, demonstrated normal performance bilaterally:

Right Ear:	5 msec threshold
Left Ear:	6 msec threshold

Audiology Extern:
Senior Staff Audiologist:

Figure 8–11.

References

Academy of Doctors of Audiology. *Code of ethics*. Retrieved February 9, 2013, from http://www.audiologist.org/academy-documents47/code-of-ethics78

American Academy of Audiology. (2011). *Code of ethics*. Retrieved February 9, 2013, from http://www.audiology.org/resources/document library/Pages/codeofethics.aspx

American National Standards Institute. (2004). *Methods for manual pure-tone threshold audiometry (ANSI S3.21-2004)*. New York, NY: Author.

American Speech and Hearing Association. (1974). Guidelines for audiometric symbols. *ASHA, 16*, 260–264.

American Speech-Language-Hearing Association. (1990). Guidelines for audiometric symbols. *ASHA, 32*(Suppl. 2), 25–30.

American Speech-Language-Hearing Association. (2010). *Code of ethics*. Retrieved February 9, 2013, from: http://www.asha.org/policy/ET 2010-00309/

Association of American Medical Colleges. (2006). *Guidelines for the use of medical interpreter services*. Retrieved February 9, 2013, from https://www.aamc.org/students/download/70338/data/interpreterguidepdf.pdf

Bennett, M. (2008). The vertigo case history. In G. Jacobson & N. Shepard (Eds.), *Balance function assessment and management*. (pp. 45–62). San Diego, CA: Plural.

Bickley, L. S., & Szilagyi, P. G. (2009). *Bates' guide to physical examination and history taking* (10th ed.). Philadelphia, PA: Wolters Kluwer Health/Lippincott Williams and Wilkins.

Blue Cross–Blue Shield of Michigan. (2005). *Provider manual chapter: Documentation guidelines for physicians and other professional providers*. Retrieved February 9, 2013 from http://ereferrals.bcbsm.com/16blue_cross_complete.pdf

Bosmans, J. M., Weyler, J. J., De Schepper, A. M., & Parizel, P. M. (2011). The radiology report as seen by radiologists and referring clinicians: Results of the COVER and ROVER surveys. *Radiology, 259*(1), 184–195.

Bunch, C. C. (1943). *Clinical audiometry.* St. Louis, MO: C. V. Mosby.

Campbell, K. C. M. (2007). *Pharmacology and ototoxicity for audiologists.* Clifton Park, NY: Thomson Delmar Learning.

Center for Medicare and Medicaid Services (2012). *Medicare benefit policy manual. Ch 15: Covered medical and other health services.* Retrieved February 9, 2013 from http://www.cms.gov/Regulations-and-Guidance/Guidance/Manuals/downloads/bp102c15.pdf

Centers for Disease Control and Prevention. (2003). HIPAA Privacy Rule and public health: Guidance from CDC and the U.S. Department of Health and Human Services. *Morbidity and Mortality Weekly Report, 52*(S–1), 1–12.

Clark, J. G., & English, K. M. (2004). *Counseling in audiologic practice: Helping patients and families adjust to hearing loss.* Boston, MA: Allyn & Bacon.

Dobie, R. A. (2002). *Medical-legal evaluation of hearing loss* (2nd ed.). San Diego, CA: Singular.

Fowler, E. P. (1930). Interpretation of audiograms. *Archives of Otolaryngology, 12*, 760–768.

Fowler, E. P. (1951). Signs, emblems and symbols of choice in plotting threshold audiograms. *Archives of Otolaryngology, 53*(2), 129–133.

Grieve, F. M., Plumb, A. A., & Khan, S. H. (2010). Radiology reporting: A general practitioner's perspective. *British Journal of Radiology, 83*, 17–22.

Hammad, A., Kysia, R., Rahab, R., Hassoun, R., & Connelly, M. (1999). *ACCESS guide to Arab culture: Health care delivery to the Arab American community.* Retrieved October 3, 2010, from http://www.access community.org/site/DocServer/health_and_research_cente_21.pdf?doc ID=381

Health Insurance Portability and Accountability Act of 1996. Pub. L. No. 104-191, 110 Stat. 1936 (1996).

Holland, A. L. (2007). *Counseling in communication disorders: A wellness perspective.* San Diego, CA: Plural.

Idowu, M. O., Bekeris, L. G., Raab, S., Ruby, S. G., & Nakhleh, R. E. (2010). Adequacy of surgical pathology reporting of cancer. *Archives of Pathology and Laboratory Medicine, 134*, 969–974.

Jacobson, G. P., & Newman, C. W. (1990). The development of the Dizziness Handicap Inventory. *Archives of Otolaryngology-Head and Neck Surgery, 116*, 424–427.

Jerger, J. (1970). Clinical experience with impedance audiometry. *Archives of Otolaryngology, 92*, 311–324.

Jerger, J. (1976). Proposed audiometric symbol system for scholarly publications. *Archives of Otolaryngology, 102,* 33–36.

Joint Committee on Infant Hearing. (2007). Year 2007 position statement: Principles and guidelines for Early Hearing Detection and Intervention programs. *Pediatrics, 120,* 898–921.

Karliner, L. S., Jacobs, E. A., Chen, A. H., & Mutha, S. (2007). Do professional interpreters improve clinical care for patients with limited English proficiency? A systematic review of the literature. *Health Services Research, 42*(2), 727–754.

Kübler-Ross, E. (1969). *On death and dying.* New York, NY: Macmillan.

Kuk, F. K., Tyler, R. S., Russell, D., & Jordan, H. (1990). The psychometric properties of a tinnitus handicap questionnaire. *Ear and Hearing, 11*(6), 434–445.

Margolis, R. H., & Saly, G. L. (2007). Toward a standard description of hearing loss. *International Journal of Audiology, 46,* 746–758.

Messenger, D. E., McLeod, R. S., & Kirsch, R. (2011). What impact has the introduction of synoptic report for rectal cancer had on reporting outcomes for specialist gastrointestinal and nongastrointestinal pathologists? *Archives of Pathology and Laboratory Medicine, 135,* 1471–1475.

Naik, S. S., Hanbridge, A., & Wilson, S. R. (2001). Radiology reports: Examining radiologist and clinician preferences regarding style and content. *American Journal of Roentgenology, 176*(3), 591–598

Newman, C. W., Jacobson, G. P., & Spitzer, J. B. (1996). Development of the tinnitus handicap inventory. *Archives of Otolaryngology-Head and Neck Surgery, 122*(2), 143–148.

Office of Minority Health. (2001). *National standards for culturally and linguistically appropriate healthcare: Final report.* Rockville, MD: Office of Minority Health, U.S. Department of Health and Human Services.

Ramachandran, V., Lewis, J. D., Mosstaghimi-Tehrnani, M., Stach, B. A., Yaremchuk, K. L. (2011). Communication outcomes in audiologic reporting. *Journal of the American Academy of Audiology, 22,* 231–241.

Roeser, R. R., & Clark, J. L. (2008). Live voice speech recognition audiometry—Stop the madness! *Audiology Today.* Jan/Feb, pp. 32–33.

Schwartz, L. H., Panicek, D. M., Berk, A. R., Li, Y., & Hricak, H. (2011). Improving communication of diagnostic radiology findings through structured reporting. *Radiology, 260*(1), 174–181.

Sierra, A. E., Bisesi, M. A., Rosenbaum, T. L., & Potchen, E. J. (1992). Readability of the radiologic report. *Investigational Radiology, 27,* 236–239.

Stach, B. A., & Ramachandran, V. (2008). Hearing disorders in children. In J. R. Madell & C. Flexer (Eds.), *Pediatric audiology: Birth through adolescence.* (pp. 3–12). New York, NY: Thieme.

The Joint Commission. (2007). *"What did the doctor say?": Improving health literacy to protect patient safety.* Oakbrook Terrace, IL: Author.

The Joint Commission. (2009). *Official "do not use" list.* Retrieved September 7, 2010, from http://www.jointcommission.org/NR/rdonlyres/2329F8F5-6EC5-4E21-B932-54B2B7D53F00/0/dnu_list.pdf

The Joint Commission. (2010). *Advancing effective communication, cultural competence, and patient- and family-centered care: A roadmap for hospitals.* Oakbrook Terrace, IL: Author.

Ventry, I. M., & Weinstein, B. E. (1982). The Hearing Handicap Inventory for the Elderly: A new tool. *Ear and Hearing, 3*(3), 128–134.

Weed, L. L. (1968). Medical records that guide and teach. *New England Journal of Medicine, 278*(11), 593–600.

Wilson-Stronks, A., & Galvez, E. (2007). *Exploring cultural and linguistic services in the nation's hospitals: A report of findings.* Oakbrook Terrace: The Joint Commission.

Wilson-Stronks, A., Lee, K. K., Cordero, C. L., Kopp, A. L., & Galvez, E. (2008). *One size does not fit all: Meeting the health care needs of diverse populations.* Oakbrook Terrace, IL: The Joint Commission.

Index

Note: Page numbers in **bold** reference non-text material.